THE DASH DIET
FOR
HYPERTENSION

Lower Your
Blood Pressure
in 14 Days—*Without Drugs*

THOMAS MOORE, M.D.,
LAURA SVETKEY, M.D., PAO-HWA LIN, PH.D.
& NJERI KARANJA, PH.D., WITH MARK JENKINS

POCKET BOOKS
New York   London   Toronto   Sydney

POCKET BOOKS, a division of Simon & Schuster, Inc.
1230 Avenue of the Americas, New York, NY 10020

ISBN 978-0-7434-1007-6

First Pocket Books printing March 2003

20 19 18 17 16 15 14

POCKET and colophon are registered trademarks of Simon & Schuster, Inc.

For information regarding special discounts for bulk purchases, please contact Simon & Schuster Special Sales at 1-800-456-6798 or business@simonandschuster.com

Cover design by Anna Dorfman

Printed in the U.S.A.

"Excellent! A medication-free alternative to help millions of Americans lower their high blood pressure and live healthier, longer lives."
—Dr. Patricia Elmer, member
Nutrition Committee, American Heart Association

ABOUT THE AUTHORS

THOMAS MOORE, M.D., has been a member of the Harvard Medical School and Boston University faculties for twenty-five years and has published more than 100 scholarly articles and book chapters on hypertension. He lives in Boston.

LAURA SVETKEY, M.D., is a professor of medicine and director of the Hypertension Center at Duke University Medical Center in Durham, North Carolina, where she lives.

PAO-HWA LIN, PH.D., has been a faculty member at the Sarah W. Stedman Nutrition Center at Duke University Medical Center since 1992. She lives in Durham.

NJERI KARANJA, PH.D., is a research scientist at the Kaiser Permanente Center for Health Research. She lives in Portland, Oregon.

MARK JENKINS is a freelance writer and the author of many successful books. He lives in Martha's Vineyard, Massachusetts.

ACKNOWLEDGMENTS

Members of the DASH Collaborative Research Group

Boston University School of Medicine: T. J. Moore

Brigham and Women's Hospital and Harvard Medical School: N. Alexander, J. Belmonte, F. Bodden, L. Cashman, P. Conlin, Y. Courtney, B. Cox, J. Dyer, A. Ghosh, J. Hackett, E. Hamilton, T. Holiday, L. Jaffe, J. Karimbakis, C. Larson, M. MacDonald, M. McCullough, D. McDonald, J. McKnight, P. McVinney, D. Moeller, T. J. Moore, P. Morris, M. Myrie, K. Nauth, K. Osborn, E. Penachio, S. Redican, F. M. Sacks, J. Sales, J. Swain, Z. Than, K. Weed;

Duke University Medical Center: J. Abbott, K. Aicher, J. Ard, C. Bales, J. Baughman, A. Bohannon, B. Brown, L. Carter, M. Drezner, R. Fike, B. Graves, K. Hoben, J. Huang, L. Johnson-Pruden, P-H. Lin, S. Norris, T. Phelps, C. Plaisted, I. Reams, P. Reams, T. Ross, F. Rukenbrod, T. Shusterman, L. P. Svetkey, E. Ward;

Johns Hopkins University: J. Abshere, L. J. Appel, D. Bengough, L. Bohlman, B. Caballero, S. Cappelli, J. Charleston, L. Clement, P. Coleman, C. Dahne, F. Dennis, S. Dobry,

K. Eldridge, T. Erlinger, A. Fouts, B. Harnish, C. Harris, B. Horseman, M. Jehn, S. Kritt, S. Kumanyika, J. Lambert, S. Lee, E. Levitas, P. McCarron, E. R. Miller, N. Muhammad, M. Nagy, B. Peterson, D. Rhodes, V. Shank, T. Shields, T. Stanger, A. Thomas, E. Thomas, R. Weiss, E. Wilke, W. Wong; *Beltsville Human Nutrition Research Center, U.S. Department of Agriculture:* S. Burns, E. Lashley, J. T. Spence;

Kaiser Permanente Center for Health Research: N. Adams, M. Aickin, M. Allison, G. Ansell, S. Baxter, N. Becker, S. Craddick, L. Diller, B. Doster, C. Eddy, D. Ernst, S. Gillespie, R. Gould, T. Haswell, L. Haworth, F. Heinith, M. Hornbrook, J. Inglish, N. Karanja, K. Kirk, P. LaChance, R. Laws, M. Leitch, W. R. Li, L. Massinger, M. McMurray, G. Meltesen, G. Miranda, S. Mitchell, J. Murphy, E. O'Connor, K. Pearson, K. Pedula, N. Redmond, J. Reinhardt, J. Rice, P. Runk, R. Schuler, C. Souvanlasy, M. Sucec, T. M. Vogt, W. M. Vollmer;

National Heart, Lung and Blood Institute: C. Brown, J. A. Cutler, M. Evans, E. Obarzanek, M. A. Proschan, D. G. Simons-Morton;

Pennington Biomedical Research Center, Louisiana State University: G. A. Bray, C. M. Champagne, S. Crawford, I. Culbert, F. Greenway, D. Harsha, J. Ihrig, B. M. Kennedy, B. McGee, E. Meador, J. Perault, D. H. Ryan, D. Sanford, A. Sawyer, S. Smith, R. Tulley, J. Vaidyanathan, M. M. Windhauser, P. J. Wozniak;

Virginia Polytechnic Institute: K. Phillips, K. K. Stewart; Washington University School of Medicine.

CONTENTS

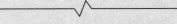

PART TWO

Making the Most of Your Commitment

PART THREE

DASH in Action

Contents

PART FOUR

DASH Menu Plans and Recipes

    Baked Catfish • Baked Macaroni and Cheese •
    BBQ Pork Chops • Blackened Beef with Greens
    and Red Potatoes • Chicken and Broccoli Bake •

PREFACE

For the first time a practical diet has been created that harnesses the blood-pressure-lowering potential of healthful foods. This diet works because it contains the amounts and combinations of key nutrients needed to lower blood pressure. It lowers blood pressure as much as most prescription blood pressure medications, and it works for men and women, whites and blacks, young and old. It is named the DASH diet after the landmark study, called "Dietary Approaches to Stop Hypertension," that proved it lowered blood pressure to a much healthier level within 14 days. The name of the diet also hints at its speed, because it is fast-acting as well as effective.

So confident are we that the DASH diet can improve your blood pressure that at the very beginning of this book we issue a "14-day challenge": we challenge you to spend two weeks eating the DASH diet—hearty meals of familiar, common foods with an emphasis on fruits, vegetables, and low-fat dairy products in a prescribed combination of servings—so you can see at the end of that time how your blood pressure has improved significantly. When you see how much it has improved, we believe you will want to continue the DASH diet for the rest of your life.

If you have been taking blood pressure medication, your doctor may eventually be able to take you off it if you're willing to remain on the DASH diet. Of course, under no circumstances should you go off your blood pressure medication without clearance from your health-care professional.

The DASH diet was developed for people who have high blood pressure (also known as hypertension), but there is a strong argument to be made that *everyone* should eat the DASH way. Blood pressure naturally goes up as you age, and the likelihood is that if you live long enough, you will eventually develop this condition (half of Americans over 65 years old have high blood pressure). Following the DASH diet enables you to halt this process.

The DASH diet is simple, but at first it may not seem easy. It involves changing eating habits you've learned over a lifetime. But the fact is that it's do-able, and in this book we provide you with all the information you need to follow the DASH way of eating. With the DASH diet you won't need a calculator every time you prepare a meal. It is based on easy-to-understand servings of whole foods, not *x* milligrams of this nutrient or *y* grams of that mineral. Simply put, we did the hard work for you.

Our focus is on nutrient-rich whole foods, instead of the nutrients themselves, making our diet available to everyone. This is not a diet just for a small group of highly motivated people who are dedicated enough to figure out how to get precise amounts of minerals and other nutrients into their diet.

The DASH Diet for Hypertension not only provides information on how the diet works but gives you sensible advice on how to make the principles of the plan part of your everyday life. If you want to take us up on our 14-day challenge, you can turn first to chapter 9, where daily menu plans will make it easy for you to start immediately on the DASH diet.

In the second half of the book, to demonstrate that healthy eating can be not just nutritious but delicious too, we have also provided 62 recipes created by our experienced nutritionists. All our recipes were taste-tested to make sure the ones we chose for this book are the very best.

Concluding the book are a number of practical resources, including a form to help you keep track of what and how much you eat. One of our goals when developing this diet was to make it easy to follow, and that includes the language we use to explain it. For those interested in more academic accounts of the DASH diet, a reading list of scientific journal articles can be found in Appendix D.

By selecting this book, you've taken a major step toward improving your health. Not only does the DASH diet treat and prevent high blood pressure, but it will reduce your risk of several deadly illnesses, including heart disease, stroke, cancer, and osteoporosis. It will also make you *feel better,* both mentally and physically. Those are not false promises but assurances based on scientific evidence.

There's nothing holding you back. So go to it. This could be the beginning of a new life dedicated to better health.

PART ONE

Why We Need DASH and How It Works

1

Introducing DASH

The Isosceles Triangle Diet. The Bacon Grease and Beer Diet. We haven't heard of either of these diets, but it wouldn't surprise us to learn they existed! No doubt about it, our society has an insatiable appetite for wonder diets that will cure all our ills—and the wackier the premise, the better. There's no reason to think people with high blood pressure are any different, especially when you consider this medical condition is so serious that it is a leading cause of heart attack, stroke, enlarged heart, and kidney damage.

If you bought this book hoping to find a blood-pressure-lowering diet with a nifty formula or handy-dandy gimmick, you'll be disappointed. The same goes if you're seeking a diet to lower your blood pressure based on some oddball theory. In a day and age when uncomplicated is unfashionable, our diet isn't high-tech or even low-tech. It's *no-tech*.

What our easy-to-understand blood-pressure-lowering diet has going for it is that not only is it safe, natural, fast-acting, and hearty enough that it won't leave you hungry, but more important, it *works*—and we have proved it.

This is no small achievement when you consider how much hype and hyperbole surround the field of health and nutrition. So many wild claims are passed off as fact. A good

Who Needs the DASH Diet?

The DASH diet is for you if you have:

- high blood pressure
- blood pressure in the "high-normal" range
- a family history of high blood pressure
- the desire to reduce your risk of heart disease, stroke, osteoporosis, and cancer
- the goal of preventing age-related high blood pressure
- a wish to get off blood pressure medications or lower your dosage
- an interest in feeling better, mentally and physically

Of course, if the above conditions apply to someone in your family or anyone close to you, then the DASH diet is for them too.

number of the diets being foisted on the American public by seemingly reputable people simply don't work, while others are plain dangerous—whether their promoters are promising to help us lose weight, live longer, or beat cancer.

Our diet to lower high blood pressure, on the other hand, was tested under carefully controlled scientific conditions. It was the subject of two of the biggest clinical research studies of their kind ever done. The studies were conducted at several of the nation's finest medical institutions under the auspices of the prestigious National Institutes of Health. More than 80 physicians, nutritionists, and technicians were involved, along with 800 study participants.

The goal was to harness the power of certain whole foods that contain the key minerals and other nutrients that we believed have the ability to lower blood pressure. This combination of nutrients had never before been tested in a "regular folks" diet.

The men and women who participated in our study followed the special diet we created. The results were beyond our wildest expectations. Our diet lowered participants' blood pressure as much as a typical blood pressure medication, and it did so quickly—within 14 days of beginning the diet. To demonstrate the effectiveness of the DASH diet, in this chapter we'll share some of the personal success stories of individual study participants.

Take Melody Smith, for example.* She is quite typical of the person with high blood pressure who participated in the DASH study. After being diagnosed with high blood pressure 10 years ago, this 42-year-old computer software salesperson tried several antihypertensive medications to keep her blood pressure down. However, Melody hated the side effects of the medications, not to mention their high cost. Sometimes she stopped taking her medications without her doctor's permission. That's when she asked us about participating in the DASH study. Melody was skeptical when she started the study but hopeful she would find a natural way to improve her blood pressure. Imagine Melody's surprise when she was informed that after just two weeks eating the DASH diet her blood pressure had dropped from 144/94 (in the "high" range) down to 132/88. The blood-pressure-lowering effect she got from the DASH diet was just about what she had gotten from the drugs she had taken before—but without the side effects. Equally important for Melody, her doctor agreed that she no longer needed to take antihypertensive medications.

The medical implications of the DASH diet are profound. If, like Melody Smith, you are one of the tens of millions of Americans with hypertension, lowering your blood pressure will enable you to significantly reduce the life-threatening consequences of this disease, including heart attack, stroke, and hardening of the arteries.

*Name and identifying characteristics changed to protect patient's identity.

The DASH Diet: A Preview of the Foods

Later in this book we explain exactly what's in the DASH diet, how the diet will lower your blood pressure, and how you can make the diet part of your daily life. We've already mentioned nutrients and how the DASH diet harnesses the power of these nutrients in a diet of whole foods, but so far we haven't told you what those foods are.

Since you're probably wondering, a preview is in order.

The DASH diet recommends that, on a daily basis, you eat about 4 servings of fruits, 4 servings of vegetables, and 2 or 3 servings of low-fat dairy foods. (For comparison, the average American diet contains only 3 or 4 servings combined of fruits and vegetables and less than one serving of dairy.) The DASH diet also includes nuts, fish, and poultry. To make "room" for these nutritious foods, the DASH diet limits fatty foods, red meat, and sugar-sweetened foods and beverages. Of course, there's much more to our diet, as you'll learn later, but the emphasis on combinations of fruits, vegetables, and low-fat dairy foods is what truly sets the DASH diet apart and makes it such an effective treatment for high blood pressure.

If your eating habits resemble those of so many Americans, without guidance you might find it a challenge to incorporate the quantities and combinations of these foods in your diet. Fortunately, you have this book to show you how.

The DASH diet will help you even if you don't have high blood pressure right now. Blood pressure tends to go up the older you get, and by their mid-sixties more than half of all Americans have high blood pressure. Following the DASH diet will help you avoid this eventuality. This is not an issue just for older people. Since blood pressure naturally starts going up in the teen years, it's almost never too early to encourage young people to start incorporating the DASH diet into their lives.

You are especially likely to develop high blood pressure if your blood pressure level is in the "high-normal" range or if you have a family history of high blood pressure. Again, eating the DASH diet can reduce the likelihood you will develop high blood pressure if you are predisposed for these reasons.

Another DASH success story is Charles Runnel, a 64-year-old retired chemistry professor. With blood pressure in the "high-normal" range (136/88), Dr. Runnel was a prime candidate for developing hypertension before he enrolled in the DASH study. Two weeks after he started eating the DASH diet, his blood pressure had dropped to 126/80. Like numerous other men and women with "high-normal" blood pressure who continued eating the DASH way after participating in the DASH study, Dr. Runnel avoided the virtual certainty he would eventually develop hypertension.

For both Melody Smith and Charles Runnel, taking medication for their blood pressure was a big issue—Melody wanted to get off her medication and Charles wanted to avoid starting one. In fact, most people who have high blood pressure are eventually prescribed medications that are often expensive and can have unpleasant and possibly harmful side effects. If you're on blood pressure medication and would like to get off or if you want to avoid ever taking medication, the DASH diet may offer more good news:

- If you have stage 1, or "mild," high blood pressure and you are not yet taking blood pressure medications, following the DASH diet could lower your blood pressure to the "healthy" range and help you avoid the possibility of ever having to take drugs for blood pressure (see the table on page 16 for classifications of the different stages of high blood pressure).

- If you are taking medications to keep your blood pressure at a healthy level and your doctor thinks you should keep taking them, following the DASH diet may help you keep your blood pressure in the healthy range on fewer medications or lower doses.
- If you have a family history of high blood pressure or "high-normal" blood pressure (again, see page 16 for classifications), the DASH diet can be an effective preventive therapy and may help you avoid ever having to take blood pressure medications.

Remember, never change your medication or stop taking a medication without first getting clearance from your doctor and having your blood pressure properly monitored.

In addition to its role in lowering blood pressure, our diet has other important benefits. The foods in the plan help to lower the risk of heart disease and osteoporosis. Surveys of the men and women who participated in our study showed that the diet actually made them feel better, physically *and* mentally. This is what the DASH diet can do for you:

- Lower your blood pressure in 14 days.
- Lower your cholesterol.
- Reduce your risk of heart disease and stroke.
- Reduce your risk of osteoporosis.
- Increase antioxidant levels in your system.
- Improve your mood and quality of life.

Above all, though, this is a diet for lowering blood pressure. Although high blood pressure is very common, it is also widely misunderstood even by those who suffer from it. Before we take a much closer look at the DASH study, it's important to learn more about the deadly disease that made this diet necessary, which we'll do in the next chapter.

Take the 14-Day DASH Diet Challenge!

We want to get you started as soon as possible on our lifesaving diet. For that reason we are issuing you our "14-day challenge." We challenge you to eat our simple diet of nutritious foods for two weeks and see the difference it makes in your blood pressure. Believe it or not, your blood pressure will drop significantly to a much healthier level.

If you have "mild" high blood pressure (stage 1), your blood pressure may go down to a level where you can go off your medication *if your doctor says it's okay.* If you have more severe high blood pressure, your blood pressure may go down to a level where you may be allowed to reduce your blood pressure medication dosage, making it easier to keep up with your drug regimen.

Sticking to the DASH diet will keep your blood pressure down, and it also has a host of other profound physical and mental health benefits, including reduced risk of heart disease, osteoporosis, and various cancers. For all these reasons, eating the DASH diet can literally save your life.

Skeptical? Don't believe a straightforward diet could have as powerful an effect as high-priced medications? *Then take the 14-day challenge!*

How do you take us up on our challenge? First, schedule an appointment with your doctor or nurse to get your blood pressure tested. Then start eating the DASH diet. At the end of 14 days, get another blood pressure reading. If you've stuck to the diet, your blood pressure will have dropped to a much healthier level. If you continue to eat the DASH diet, your blood pressure will stay at a healthy level.

Why are we so confident your blood pressure will respond? Because we achieved these results in hundreds of men and women who participated in the DASH study.

Caution

Keep in mind, the 14-day challenge may not be for everyone. Some people with kidney problems may not tolerate the amount of potassium contained in DASH foods. If this applies to you, talk to your doctor before starting the diet. But for most people the DASH diet is a healthy eating plan that has been proven to lower blood pressure. For guidance on easing into the DASH diet, refer to page 146.

And remember our admonition to get clearance from your doctor before making any change in your medication regimen.

2

Why DASH?
Hypertension: The Silent Killer

An astounding one in four adult Americans suffers from hypertension—50 million of our citizens in all. The presence of this condition is even more widespread among older Americans, more than half of whom have hypertension. Despite its prevalence, hypertension is seriously underestimated. To understand how deadly this disease is, just consider that it is a prime risk factor for both heart disease and stroke, the first and third leading causes of death in this country, and is responsible for one-quarter of all cases of kidney failure in the United States. High blood pressure can also cause other life-threatening problems. Bottom line: If you have hypertension, you need to deal with it, or it may kill you.

Before we go any further, a word about terminology. The two terms *hypertension* and *high blood pressure* can be used interchangeably, although we use *high blood pressure* much more often.

A Deadly Disease That Affects Millions

About 50 million Americans suffer from hypertension. Medicine has made a lot of progress in the fight against this disease, but we are a long way from where we need to be. Consider these statistics on conditions that are caused by high blood pressure:

- Stroke rates are up slightly since 1993.
- The society-wide improvement in heart disease is slowing.
- The prevalence of kidney failure requiring dialysis or transplantation is increasing.
- The prevalence of congestive heart failure is increasing.

If you have hypertension, you do not experience pain or other noticeable symptoms for many years. The only way you can tell you have hypertension is to be tested for it. About one-third of people with high blood pressure don't even know they have it and therefore do not seek treatment. Even those who *do* get attention for their high blood pressure frequently discontinue treatment because it doesn't make them feel any better. Only half of those people with hypertension are taking medication, and only about a quarter have their high blood pressure under control.

However, if untreated, hypertension can lead to a host of serious and possibly life-threatening medical problems (see page 17). Seemingly benign and yet so deadly, hypertension has been called the silent killer.

What Is High Blood Pressure/Hypertension?

Each time your heart beats, it pumps out blood through your arteries. "Blood pressure" is the force of the blood pushing against the walls of your arteries, which deliver blood throughout your body.

Your blood pressure is at its greatest when the heart contracts to pump out blood. This is called *systolic* pressure. Your blood pressure falls when the heart is at rest between beats. This is called *diastolic* pressure.

Different activities make your blood pressure go up or down. For example, running to catch the bus will increase your blood pressure. On the other hand, when you're asleep, your blood pressure is relatively low. Such changes in blood pressure are normal.

Some people have blood pressure that is high all or most of the time. Their blood constantly pushes against the walls of their arteries with higher than normal force. These people have a condition called hypertension. High blood pressure is dangerous because it makes your heart work harder and damages your blood vessels.

What Causes High Blood Pressure?

The majority of people who have hypertension are predisposed to the disease because it runs in their family. However, some people who are not predisposed to hypertension may develop the disease simply because of poor diet and lifestyle.

Whether or not you have a genetic tendency, your chances of developing high blood pressure are much greater under the following circumstances:

- You eat very little fruit, vegetables, or low-fat dairy products.
- Your diet is high in salt.
- You are overweight.
- You drink a lot of alcohol.
- You rarely or never exercise.

Conversely, even if you have a family history of hypertension, a healthy diet and lifestyle may protect you against developing it.

America's High-Priced Diet

The American diet is responsible for a major portion of the U.S. health-care price tag, estimated to be over $1 trillion. The following are some of the costs that could be reduced by widespread adoption of the DASH diet:

Cardiovascular disease: Coronary heart disease and strokes cost $128 billion in treatment and lost productivity.

Cancer: More than $104 billion is spent for cancer, including treatment, lost productivity, and mortality costs.

Diabetes mellitus: Annually $92 billion, including direct and indirect costs, is spent on diabetes care.

Who Is Most at Risk for Hypertension?

Some people are more likely to develop high blood pressure than others. For example, high blood pressure is more common in African-Americans than in whites, and it develops earlier and is more severe in African-Americans.

There are also gender differences. In the early and middle adult years, men are more likely to have high blood pressure than women. But as men and women age, the reverse becomes true. More women after menopause have high blood pressure than men of the same age. And the number of both men and women with high blood pressure increases rapidly in older age groups. More than half of all Americans over age 65 have high blood pressure.

As already described, heredity can make some people more likely than others to develop high blood pressure. If your parents or grandparents had high blood pressure, your risk may be increased. While high blood pressure is mainly a disease of adults, it can occur in children as well. Indeed, with children in our society eating less healthy diets and becoming less active physically and more overweight, high blood pressure in children is on the rise.

Addressing Hypertension:
It's Never Too Early to Start

Blood pressure usually starts off normal in childhood and rises gradually as we get older. But blood pressure goes up higher and faster in some people depending on their diet, lifestyle, and whether they are predisposed to developing hypertension. Unless predisposed individuals take preventive measures, eventually they develop blood pressure that is defined as "high." Because the trend toward high blood pressure starts in adolescence, the ideal time to address this problem is in childhood. Doing so is an effective way to slow the rise in blood pressure so that it never reaches the "high" range. If your children have a family history of high blood pressure, then the earlier they start eating the DASH diet and taking other measures to lower their blood pressure, the better their chance of never developing the disease.

Understanding Blood Pressure Readings

Blood pressure readings tell us what our systolic and diastolic pressures are, with one number on top of the other and the top number always being the systolic pressure. An example of a blood pressure reading is 120/80 mm Hg (millimeters of mercury), which you would say as "120 over 80." This means your systolic blood pressure is 120 mm Hg and your diastolic blood pressure is 80 mm Hg.

A blood pressure less than 130/85 mm Hg is considered normal, and a blood pressure below 120/80 mm Hg is considered even better for your heart and blood vessels. It was once believed that low blood pressure (such as 105/65 mm Hg in an adult) was harmful. However, except in rare cases, even very low blood pressure is healthy.

Alert: There is growing evidence that not only is having "high-normal" blood pressure (130–140/85–90) a risk factor for eventually developing severe high blood pressure, but the medical problems caused by high blood pressure—particularly those that lead to stroke and heart disease—begin when blood pressure is in this high-normal range. This reinforces the need to be vigilant about your blood pressure even when it isn't, strictly speaking, "high."

High blood pressure, or hypertension (above 140 systolic and/or above 90 diastolic), is classified by stages and is more serious as the numbers get higher. The following table shows the most up-to-date system doctors use to classify people's blood pressure:

Condition	Systolic Pressure	Diastolic Pressure	What to Do
Normal	Less than 130	Less than 85	Recheck in 2 years
High-normal	130–140	85–90	Recheck in 1 year
Hypertension			
Stage 1	140–159	90–99	See doctor within 2 months
Stage 2	160–179	100–109	See doctor within 1 month
Stage 3	180 and up	110 and up	See doctor within 1 week

Truth and Consequences

Although high blood pressure usually has no *noticeable* symptoms, the consequences are deadly serious and include the following:

Arteriosclerosis ("hardening of the arteries"): High blood pressure harms the arteries by making them thick and stiff. This accelerates the buildup of cholesterol and fats in the blood vessels, which clog the vessels like rust in a pipe. This in turn prevents the blood from flowing through the body and in time can lead to heart attack or stroke.

Heart attack: Blood carries oxygen to the body. When the arteries that bring blood to the heart become blocked, the heart muscle does not get enough oxygen. Reduced blood flow can cause chest pain (angina). Eventually the flow may be stopped completely, causing a portion of heart muscle to suffer irreversible injury—or heart attack.

Stroke: A stroke is a "brain attack." When high blood pressure narrows the blood vessels to the brain, less blood can get to the brain. If one of the narrowed arteries gets blocked completely, the part of the brain fed by that artery doesn't get enough oxygen and nourishment, and a stroke (thrombotic stroke) may occur. A stroke can also occur when very high pressure causes a break in a weakened blood vessel in the brain (hemorrhagic stroke).

Enlarged heart: High blood pressure causes the heart to work harder. Over time this causes the heart to thicken and stretch. Eventually the heart fails to pump normally, causing fluids to back up into the lungs, a condition called congestive heart failure.

Kidney damage: The kidney acts as a filter to rid the body of extra fluid and wastes. Over a number of years, high blood pressure can narrow and thicken the blood vessels of the kidney. When this happens, the kidney filters less fluid, and waste builds up in the blood. The kidneys may fail altogether. When this happens, medical treatment (dialysis) or a kidney transplant may be needed.

High Blood Pressure Medications

There are several types of medications for controlling high blood pressure. Sometimes a doctor has to prescribe different drugs to find the one that works best for you. Sometimes more than one drug is necessary. The following are some of the various blood pressure medications:

Diuretics, sometimes called water pills: Eliminate excess water and salt from the body (popular names: Diuril, Hydrodiuril, chlorthalidone,hydrochlorothiazide).

Beta blockers: Reduce the heart rate and the output of blood by counteracting a hormone called noradrenaline (popular names: Tenormin, Lopressor, Inderal, atenolol, metoprolol, propranolol).

Angiotensin converting enzyme (ACE) inhibitors: Interfere with the production of angiotensin, a chemical that causes arteries to constrict (popular names: Vasotec, Prinivil, Capoten, enalapril, lisinopril, captopril).

Calcium channel blockers: Relax the blood vessels (popular brand names: Procardia, diltiazem, amlodipine, verapamil).

Vasodilators: Cause the vessels to dilate, thus relaxing their walls and lowering blood pressure (popular name: hydralazine).

Central nervous system agents: Prevent the brain from sending impulses that stimulate blood vessels to constrict and raise blood pressure (popular names: Aldomet, alphamethyldopa).

Angiotensin II inhibitors: Block the binding of angiotensin to the arteries (popular names: Cozaar, Diovan, Avapro).

Controlling high blood pressure can prevent all these conditions from developing.

How High Blood Pressure Is Treated

If you have *mild* hypertension, you may be able to bring your blood pressure into the healthy range by cutting down on salty foods, exercising and losing weight, and drinking alcohol in moderation. But sticking with these measures can be a challenge, and most people require medications to be successful in lowering blood pressure. For moderate and severe high blood pressure, antihypertensive medications are almost always required. While effective, these drugs can be expensive and may have unpleasant side effects, such as fatigue, weakness, light-headedness, headache, digestive problems, and sexual dysfunction.

What has been missing is an approach to treating hypertension that is simple, safe, and effective. Some of us have long believed there is such a way to treat hypertension. We think an important factor affecting blood pressure has been neglected during the quest for hypertension treatments and that, if it were properly looked into, a breakthrough in treating hypertension would be possible.

What is that factor? It is, quite simply, *the proper diet.* Specifically, certain foods, when eaten in the right amounts and combinations, have the ability to lower blood pressure significantly. These foods are the focus of the DASH diet.

3

Proving the Diet Works:
How We Did It

For about a quarter century many of us in medicine believed that the way hypertension was treated didn't fully take into consideration a major factor: the change in the modern Western diet during the past century. After all, the rise in the incidence of hypertension and other chronic diseases has occurred in conjunction with a *decline* in our consumption of fruits and vegetables and grains and a dramatic *increase* in how much salt, sugar, fat, and cholesterol we eat.

In the rest of the world, populations who eat a diet similar to that of our ancestors tend to have healthy blood pressure. People who live in remote, non-Westernized areas and vegetarians comprise two groups whose diet more closely resembles the one our forebears ate than the one we eat today, and they tend to have a low incidence of hypertension. We doctors and nutritionists specializing in hypertension began to wonder why. It became apparent that high amounts of particular minerals in their diets seemed to lower blood pressure, although the evidence wasn't always consistent; the minerals eventually identified were potassium, magnesium, and calcium. Non-mineral nutrients whose presence (or absence) might be affecting their blood pressure were fiber and protein (beneficial) and fat (harmful).

What Is a "Diet"?

The word *diet* refers to the way we eat, whatever that is. Too many people think a "diet" is a plan we follow temporarily to achieve a short-term goal—usually to shed a few pounds and look better in a swimsuit. If we are reducing calories to lose weight, that's a "weight-loss" diet. If we don't eat meat, that's a "vegetarian" diet. If all we eat is soda and snack foods, that's a "junk food" diet. The DASH diet, of course, is an eating system designed to lower blood pressure. But it's balanced in all the major food groups and is consistent with the eating patterns recommended by nutritionists for almost everyone. That's why we think of it as the DASH diet for hypertension—and for life.

Researchers tried to discover the precise quantities of potassium, magnesium, and calcium that people with high blood pressure needed to consume to lower their blood pressure. So in study after study, volunteers were given mineral supplements in pill form and the effects on their blood pressure were carefully recorded. Some studies used individual minerals, while others used combinations of minerals. Other studies attempted to determine the effect on blood pressure of varying the amount of fat, protein, and fiber in the diet.

Nothing worked consistently. Sometimes participants' blood pressure readings went down; sometimes they didn't. The process was frustrating, the goal elusive.

Top-Level Study Finally Launched

So important a health-care issue is hypertension and so great a need is there for an effective way to treat it that in 1992 the National Institutes of Health stepped in. Promising funds for research, the government-run NIH put out the call for a team of doctors and nutritionists who believed they could find a way to treat hypertension by focusing on the role of key nutrients in the diet. This would not be any ordinary study—the top brass at the National Institutes for Health, which oversees the National Heart, Lung, and Blood Institute, wanted it to be the biggest, best, and most conclusive research of its kind done in this field.

We were the team the NHLBI selected for the mammoth task of finding a proven way to treat hypertension using key nutrients. Drawn from five top medical facilities—Harvard, Duke, Johns Hopkins, Pennington Biomedical Research Center, and the Center for Health Research at Kaiser Permanente—our number included dozens of physicians, nutritionists, statisticians, nurses, and research coordinators.

Although our intention was to design a study that would show how to use all the key nutrients to lower blood pressure, this time the focus would be on getting these nutrients in a diet of *real foods*, not in handfuls of pills. Given the failure of mineral supplement studies, our theory was that there might be something about consuming certain minerals in a diet of real foods that would more reliably lower blood pressure than consuming mineral supplements in pill form—partly because our bodies are more efficient at using minerals when they are consumed in whole food form and also because the minerals may interact with other components in whole foods to do their job better. We also considered the possibility that the key nutrients that affect blood pressure (minerals, as well as fiber, protein, and fat) need to be consumed in quite specific combinations to lower blood pressure effectively. These ideas became the premise of our investigation. How we intended to prove it was in a rigorous scientific study that no one would ever be able to dispute, one that was soon given the name Dietary Approaches to Stop Hypertension, or DASH for short.

DASH Study Design

The results of the DASH study are taken seriously because of the way we conducted the research. What we did was perform a "carefully controlled clinical trial"—medical language for a foolproof way to test a treatment—that featured both a large number of participants and close monitoring, two factors that ensure accurate results.

More than 8,800 people volunteered for the DASH study.

DASH—Just Another Study?

So many study results are reported in the media that it's difficult to know which ones to take seriously. The DASH diet is treated with great respect in many quarters for several reasons, including:

- The study was supported and sponsored by the prestigious National Institutes of Health.
- The diet was tested at several of the world's most respected medical institutions.
- A large number of participants enrolled in the study.
- The study participants varied in age, gender, race, and socioeconomic group.
- The study participants were carefully monitored.
- The study and its results were reviewed by a panel of experts who recommended it for publication in the prestigious *New England Journal of Medicine*.
- The diet is recommended by the American Heart Association and several other esteemed medical organizations.
- The DASH diet is now part of the official high blood pressure guidelines here in the U.S. and abroad.

Why Test the DASH Diet on People Who Don't Have Hypertension?

When we tested the DASH diet, we included people both with and without hypertension. Why bother testing the diet on people with normal blood pressure levels? The reason is simple. People with blood pressure that is in the "high-normal" range are at greater risk of heart attack and stroke than those who have ideal blood pressure. Also, those with high-normal blood pressure frequently end up developing hypertension, and lowering their blood pressure would prevent that from happening.

From this number, 459 were chosen to participate. Some of the participants had high blood pressure and some did not. These men and women were drawn from the communities around the four medical facilities where the research took place: Boston, Massachusetts (Harvard Medical School); Baltimore, Maryland (Johns Hopkins Medical School); Durham, North Carolina (Duke University Medical School); and Baton Rouge, Louisiana (Pennington Biomedical Research Center).

The average age of the participants was 46, and the average blood pressure reading was 132/85. Almost 60 percent of the participants were African-American, and 49 percent were women. Those using hypertension medications were weaned off their drugs so that the effects of test diets could be precisely measured.

The study was divided into two parts. There was a preliminary three-week period when all 459 participants ate a "typical American diet." This was done to get all the participants to the same nutritional status.

Following this preliminary phase, the participants were randomly assigned to one of three different diets for eight weeks:

- a continuation of the typical American diet
- a diet similar to the typical American diet, but with more fruits and vegetables
- the DASH diet—rich in fruits, vegetables, and low-fat dairy products; moderate in fish, poultry, and nuts; and reduced in red meat, sweets, and sugar-sweetened drinks

To help them stick with their particular diets, we fed the participants their main meal of the day at their local study center (those living in the Baltimore area, for instance, ate lunch or dinner at Johns Hopkins). The rest of the day's meals were prepackaged and consumed by the participants elsewhere. Every day we had all 459 participants fill out a short checklist that helped us keep track of allowed beverages (up

---

The Significance of Salt

The issue of salt is an important one. Salt is known to contribute to high blood pressure. However, because we wanted to focus on the effects of whole foods when we conducted the DASH study, we didn't make any of the diets "low salt." In spite of this, the DASH diet lowered blood pressure significantly. This proves that a diet high in vegetables, fruits, and low-fat dairy is an effective treatment for high blood pressure—even when it isn't low in salt.

In a follow-up study called DASH-Sodium, we proved that the DASH diet combined with a reduction in salt was even more effective at lowering blood pressure. The bottom line is that the DASH diet will work to lower your blood pressure even if you don't make it low salt, but you can optimize the effectiveness of the DASH diet by reducing the amount of salt in it (see chapter 4, "Optimizing the Diet: Salt Reduction Is the Answer").

to three servings daily of coffee, tea, or diet soft drinks and up to two alcoholic drinks), salt/sodium intake, consumption of any nonpermitted foods, and omission of study foods. We also had the study participants provide periodic urine samples to confirm that they had eaten more than 90 percent of the food provided—a statistic that would make for an extremely accurate study.

We had to make sure the participants weren't doing anything else that might lower their blood pressure. They were asked not to make any major changes in their level of physical activity during the study. We weighed the participants frequently to make sure they stayed the weight they were when the study began; if someone gained or lost a few pounds, we gave them a bit less or more food to eat to get their weight back to what it was. Salt/sodium intake was the same in all three diets—slightly lower than the U.S. average but still higher than what most guidelines recommended.

To prevent bias, we were not allowed to see or know the results of the study until it was completed (in scientific terms, we were "blinded"). That meant that because the DASH study began in 1994, it was 1996 before we knew whether we had been successful or not. However, when we saw the results, we knew it had been worth the wait.

The Results

We tested the effects of three different diets: the so-called typical American diet, a diet rather like the typical American diet but with large added amounts of fruits and vegetables, and the DASH diet.

Those who ate the typical American diet did not see a change in their blood pressure. Those on the fruit and vegetable diet experienced a significant lowering of their systolic blood pressure—the upper number that is a measurement of blood pressure in the arteries when the heart contracts to

Results of the DASH Study in Participants with High Blood Pressure

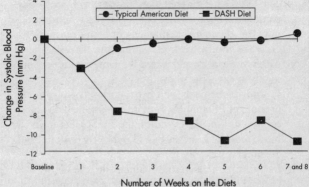

The beneficial effects of the DASH diet on people with high blood pressure (hypertensives) are even more impressive when represented visually. As you can see in the above graph, systolic blood pressure readings for hypertensives who ate the typical American diet during the DASH study stayed about the same, while people who ate the DASH diet for the eight-week period experienced a significant and rapid lowering of their systolic blood pressure. In participants with high blood pressure, systolic blood pressure dropped an average of 11.4 mm Hg during the DASH study.

pump out blood—but little change in their diastolic pressure.

The results of the DASH diet, however, were truly extraordinary. The men and women who ate the DASH diet for eight weeks experienced a significant drop in both their systolic *and* diastolic blood pressure readings. Changes occurred within a week of starting the diet, stabilized within two weeks, and stayed lowered for the remainder of the eight weeks (see graph). On average, blood pressure fell 5.5 mm Hg (systolic) and 3.0 mm Hg (diastolic) among all participants in our study. In participants with high blood pressure (systolic blood pressure of 140 mm Hg or more or diastolic blood pressure of 90

The DASH Study: Results at a Glance

- The DASH diet lowered blood pressure in DASH study participants by an average of 5.5 mm Hg (systolic) and 3 mm Hg (diastolic). Reductions in blood pressure occurred within a week of starting the diet, stabilized within two weeks, and stayed the same for the remaining six weeks of the study.
- In study participants with hypertension (systolic blood pressure of 140 mm Hg or more or diastolic blood pressure of 90 mm Hg or more), the DASH diet lowered blood pressure an average of 11.4 mm Hg (systolic) and 5.5 mm Hg (diastolic).
- In African-American study participants, the DASH diet lowered blood pressure an average of 6.9 mm Hg (systolic) and 3.3 mm Hg (diastolic).
- The DASH diet lowered cholesterol in study participants an average of 7 percent (14 cholesterol points).
- The DASH diet lowered homocysteine in the blood 7 to 9 percent (elevated homocysteine levels are associated with heart disease and stroke).

mm Hg or more), the results were even more dramatic: blood pressure dropped an average of 11.4 mm Hg (systolic) and 5.5 mm Hg (diastolic). These improvements were the same as those achieved using standard blood pressure medications.

There were positive health outcomes of the DASH diet beyond lowering high blood pressure. Most important, perhaps, the DASH diet lowered the study participants' cholesterol levels. When blood cholesterol is high, cholesterol and other fatty substances collect on the walls of blood vessels and in time restrict or block the flow of blood to the heart. High cholesterol, which is generally caused by a diet high in saturated fats, is a major risk factor for heart disease. The DASH diet is

DASH and Insulin Levels

Many people worry that eating carbohydrates (sugar, bread, and starchy vegetables like potatoes) will increase the insulin level in their bloodstream and that a high insulin level will contribute to the development of hardening of the arteries, diabetes, mood changes, and weight gain (by stimulating hunger). While DASH is a carbohydrate-rich eating pattern, it contains very little true sugar, or what we call simple sugar. Simple sugars—like those in candy, cookies, or granulated sugar—are rapidly absorbed by the digestive system and cause sudden increases in blood sugar and insulin levels. The carbohydrates in DASH are "complex" (as opposed to simple) and are digested slowly, causing less abrupt changes in blood sugar and insulin.

We measured blood sugar and insulin levels very carefully and precisely in the DASH study participants to see if this was an issue. We found that those on the DASH diet had no differences in blood sugar or insulin levels compared to the participants who were eating a typical American diet. And so we determined that there is no reason to be concerned that the carbohydrates contained in DASH diet foods pose any kind of insulin-related risk.

low in total fat and saturated fat, and in people who ate the diet during the study, cholesterol dropped 7 percent (14 cholesterol points).

Another notable feature of the DASH diet was that it lacked harmful or unpleasant side effects. There was no downside to the DASH diet, except for a very small number of study participants who suffered from mild gastrointestinal upset (gas and loose stools), which resolved itself as soon as they got used to the increased amounts of healthy fruits and vegetables in their diet.

The Science Behind DASH

"Yes, but how does it *work?*" That's the question we often hear once people learn how effective the DASH diet is in treating hypertension.

As scientists, we have proved that the diet works; what we cannot prove is exactly why it works. Therefore, the short answer to that oft-asked question is "We don't know." We designed the DASH diet to be especially rich in several key nutrients— minerals like potassium, calcium, and magnesium, for example—which have been suggested to help lower blood pressure. But we "prescribe" these nutrients as whole foods, and whole foods contain hundreds of substances that may be equally important in providing the blood pressure effect of the DASH diet. It may be that the combined nutrients in the DASH foods work together to create an effect greater than the sum of their parts. Indeed, it is virtually impossible to measure the specific effect of an individual nutrient on blood pressure when it is delivered in a diet of whole foods rather than a pill. For example, if you want to test whether magnesium is effective in lowering blood pressure, you might increase a person's consumption of nuts, but nuts are also high in fiber and potassium, which are believed to lower blood pressure too.

What we do know is that *together*, in certain combinations and when eaten as part of a whole-food diet, DASH foods are successful in lowering blood pressure to much healthier levels. As scientists, we avoid making claims we can't support with proof. That said, we *can* make educated guesses based on the available evidence and tell you why we think certain minerals and nutrients help keep your blood pressure healthy.

Those of you who are interested in the science behind DASH can refer to Appendix A, which provides some interesting and informative background on this fascinating subject.

Implications of the Diet

Now that you've seen what went into creating the DASH diet, it's worth summarizing what our eating plan can do to change your life.

If you have high blood pressure, getting your blood pressure to a healthier level will help you avoid a host of potentially life-threatening diseases—in particular, heart disease and stroke. Experts agree that widespread adoption of the DASH diet by Americans would result in a 15 percent decrease in coronary heart disease in our population and a 27 percent reduction in the number of strokes. Unlike any of the "fad diets" currently on the market, the DASH diet is endorsed by several distinguished medical organizations, including the American Heart Association.

But the DASH diet is more than a treatment for people who already have high blood pressure. It also prevents high blood pressure from eventually occurring in people predisposed to this condition because of a family history of hyper-

---

Antioxidants and the DASH Diet

Antioxidants are compounds in foods that can help slow down or prevent certain chronic health problems, including heart disease, cancer, and stroke. The DASH diet is high in antioxidant-rich foods, such as fruits and vegetables, whole grains, nuts, and vegetable oils.

In tests of DASH diet study participants, we found that eating the DASH diet increased their levels of specific antioxidants (beta carotene, lutein, cryptozanthin, and zeaxanthin).

The high amount of antioxidants in DASH foods is another reason to start eating the DASH way.

tension or because they have blood pressure in the "high-normal" range. Keep in mind, too, that because blood pressure naturally rises with age (over half of Americans over 65 have high blood pressure), starting to eat the DASH way can help prevent this eventuality.

If you eat the DASH diet, you will also reduce your risk of getting cancer, because a diet rich in fruits, vegetables, and grains is known to reduce the risk of this killer condition. The DASH diet is completely compatible with the nutrient recommendations of the American Cancer Society.

And because it is rich in calcium, the DASH diet can help you avoid developing osteoporosis, a bone-thinning disease that affects millions of Americans, both men and women.

A "Feel-Good" Diet Too!

Very few studies have used scientific methods to investigate the effects of dietary changes on quality of life. A substudy of DASH looked into this very issue. The results strongly reinforced the benefits of eating the DASH diet.

We assessed our study participants' quality of life before and after the eight-week study period, using a detailed questionnaire that asked participants about several areas of their quality of life. Questions included "How much does your physical health interfere with your work or daily life?" and "How energetic do you feel most of the time?"

People who ate the DASH diet for eight weeks during the study reported feeling better at the end than before starting the diet. Their quality of life *improved*, according to the positive responses they gave to much of the nine-part questionnaire. The fact that participants didn't report feeling the same or worse is extremely important from our point of view and is, from the perspective of nutritional scientists, a "big deal."

Thus, the DASH diet can actually make you feel better.

Partly that is because it is not a low-calorie eating plan—you don't feel deprived and "grumpy" because of it. But just as important, the presence of plenty of key nutrients in the DASH diet is health promoting, and it's only natural that we are happier when this is the case.

A Postmodern Diet

Despite all the extraordinary progress we have made in medicine, science, and technology, the changes in our diet over the last couple of generations have spelled health disaster. The modern American diet is responsible for a host of killer illnesses, including heart disease, stroke, cancer, and osteoporosis. We will probably never eradicate all these diseases, but we can take a single major step toward preventing them. Surgeon General Everett Koop put it succinctly in 1988: "One personal choice seems to influence long-term health more than any other: *what we eat.*"

We need to return to the kind of eating plan that seems to suit the human body best. A fiber-rich whole-food diet that emphasizes fruits, vegetables, and low-fat dairy foods will benefit virtually everyone, but it has special implications for people with high blood pressure.

The DASH diet is precisely that kind of diet.

PART TWO

Making the Most of
Your Commitment

4

Optimizing the Diet:
Salt Reduction Is the Answer

The focus of the DASH study was a whole-food diet rich in the key nutrients that we believed would significantly improve blood pressure health. We were aware that for DASH to be an accurate study of the diet itself we would have to minimize the impact of certain factors known to lower blood pressure—particularly exercise, alcohol restriction, and weight loss. So we asked participants not to exercise more or less than they usually did and not to alter their alcohol intake, and we weighed participants regularly and adjusted their calorie intake accordingly if they gained or lost weight.

Our most significant decision, though, was to eliminate the role salt might play in the study. We did this by making sure the salt content in all three of the diets we tested was the same and also by not making the diets "low salt." Our main reason for not making DASH a low-salt diet was so we could be sure it was the nutrient-rich whole foods that produced the outcome we were measuring, not the effects of a reduced salt content. We also wanted to create a foundation for our eating plan that emphasized what people need to get *more of* in their diet to make them healthier—in this case fruits, vegetables, and low-fat dairy foods—not what they should limit. And, of course, we proved this to be effective.

Salt, Sodium . . . What's the Connection?

Most of us know there's a connection between salt and sodium, but we don't know exactly what it is. Sodium and chloride are the two chemical ingredients in salt. Sodium is the chemical that regulates the amount of fluid in our bodies and, to some extent, blood pressure. Table salt is made up of approximately 40 percent sodium, so 1 gram of salt (1,000 milligrams) contains 400 milligrams of sodium.

The DASH-Sodium Study

The medical profession has long believed that a salty diet contributes to high blood pressure, and several studies have shown that reducing salt intake lowers blood pressure in most people. Soon after the results of the DASH study came in, we launched a study to test whether the DASH diet would work even better if it was low in salt. We called the study DASH-Sodium.

The results of DASH-Sodium have been incorporated into the recommendations of this book. First, the results confirmed what so many of us had long suspected but which numerous scientists before us had not been able to prove definitively—that a diet low in salt *does* lower blood pressure. Second, the results demonstrated that a low-salt version of the DASH diet (with 3.8 grams of salt a day) produced a greater blood-pressure-lowering effect than the DASH diet by itself (with 7 grams of salt a day).

DASH-Sodium study participants who ate the low-salt version of the DASH diet experienced a 9-point drop in their blood pressure, as compared to a drop of 6 points after eating the DASH diet without salt reduction. The beneficial effects of eating the low-salt DASH-Sodium diet were the greatest in

DASH-Sodium Study: Results at a Glance

The recently completed DASH-Sodium study tested the DASH diet with and without salt reduction to see if the two approaches combined worked better than either alone. Key results include:

- On their own, the DASH diet and a low-salt version of a typical American diet each lowered blood pressure, but blood pressure dropped to even healthier levels in people who ate a combination of these two diets (i.e., a low-salt version of the DASH diet).
- The low-salt version of the DASH diet lowered blood pressure in study participants with both normal and high blood pressure, but the diet was especially effective in people with high blood pressure.
- African-American study participants experienced especially significant reductions in blood pressure.

   The version of the DASH diet that produced these results had a sodium content of about 1,500 milligrams per day, half that of the "typical American diet" used as a comparison in the same study.

people who had high blood pressure—the diet reduced their blood pressure by an average of almost 12 points.

The results of DASH-Sodium are quite extraordinary and represent a powerful way to optimize the DASH diet. More so than the original DASH diet, the low-salt DASH diet may enable you to go off your medication or lower your dosage (only with your doctor's clearance). Widespread adoption of the low-salt DASH diet could make it possible for additional millions of Americans already eating the DASH diet to lower their dosages further or altogether stop taking medications that are often expensive and have unpleasant and potentially harmful side effects.

DASH-Sodium lays to rest any remaining questions about whether reducing salt intake does in fact lower blood pressure. The study was held at the same prestigious medical institutions as the original clinical trial. And like its landmark predecessor, DASH-Sodium was a large, carefully controlled study engaging a diverse group of 412 study participants who followed a tightly monitored feeding regimen. The study found that the low-salt version of the DASH diet lowered blood pressure in all the subgroups of study participants— those with normal and high blood pressure, men and women, black and white, young and old.

Because reducing the salt content of the DASH diet made it significantly better at lowering blood pressure, all the recipes given in chapter 10 were developed with a reduced salt content to maximize their blood pressure effectiveness for you.

How Salt Influences Blood Pressure

Although salt has a bad name, the fact is that it is an essential part of everyone's diet and you couldn't live without it. The main ingredient in salt is sodium. You cannot exist without sodium, but the amount you need is very small, less than 1 gram per day. Yet the average American eats a daily diet with about 10 grams of salt in it (4 grams of sodium), and many of us eat up to 15 grams a day (6 grams of sodium).

Ten grams of salt is almost 2 teaspoonfuls. You probably don't add that much salt to your food from your saltshaker. Most of the salt in our diets is found in the processed foods that have become a ubiquitous part of the modern American diet. "Hidden" sources of salt include bread, processed meat, cheese, canned vegetables—the list is endless. Trouble is, we can't remove the salt from these foods when we eat them by

themselves or use them for cooking. Government food-labeling regulations help us monitor the sodium content in processed foods. However, in restaurant foods—especially from fast-food chains and Chinese and Mexican restaurants—the sodium levels can be very high.

Certain people are especially vulnerable to developing high blood pressure if they eat a too-salty diet. Slightly less than half of people with high blood pressure are "salt sensitive"—that is, salt intake is more likely to increase their blood pressure, and salt restriction more likely to lower it. There is no simple "test" we can do to identify people who are salt-sensitive, but those most likely to be are overweight, older, and African-American. Of course, people not in those groups can be salt-sensitive as well. A low-salt diet is of special benefit to anyone who is salt-sensitive.

We think salt increases blood pressure because, when you eat a lot of salt, the presence of sodium in your blood attracts a lot of water and causes fluid retention. Extra fluid in your system expands the volume of blood in your blood vessels, puts pressure on the walls of the vessels, and increases blood pressure.

Lowering Your Salt/Sodium Intake: Here's How

Up until now we've talked mostly about salt in this chapter. Now we're going to talk about sodium because we are going to teach you how to read food labels, which report sodium content. In line with government recommendations, food labels suggest you limit your sodium intake to 2,400 milligrams of sodium a day. However, the DASH-Sodium study found that it is better for your blood pressure if you eat a little less salt than that amount—preferably between 1,500 and 2,000 milligrams a day.

One of the most important ways to reduce your sodium in-

Macaroni & Cheese

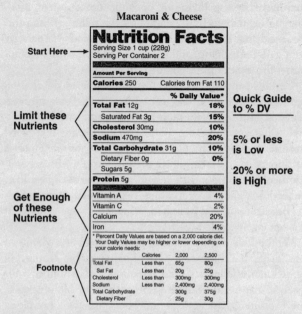

take is to learn to understand the Nutrition Facts panel on food packaging so you will know how to choose foods low in salt. Studies show that people who pay attention to the Nutrition Facts panel are healthier than those who ignore it.

To find out whether the food you are looking at on the

	% **Daily Value***
Total Fat 12g	**18%**
Saturated Fat 3g	**15%**
Cholesterol 30mg	**10%**
Sodium 470mg	**20%**

supermarket shelf is high, low, or moderate in sodium content, you need to focus on the "% Daily Value" column of numbers on the right-hand side of the Nutrition Facts panel.

If the % Daily Value for sodium is 5 or less, the food is considered low in sodium; higher than 20 and it is considered high in that nutrient. To keep the sodium in your diet to a minimum, your goal should be to select, as often as possible, foods that have a % Daily Value for sodium of 5 or less.

Here are some other tips to help you reduce your sodium intake:

- Look for products that say "sodium free," "very low sodium," "low sodium," "light in sodium," "reduced or less sodium," or "unsalted." Because the government has implemented strict rules to govern such claims, you can be assured these are not empty promises.
- Buy fresh or plain frozen vegetables. Canned vegetables are okay if labeled "no salt added." Use fresh poultry, fish, and lean meat rather than canned or processed versions.
- Use herbs, spices, and salt-free seasoning blends in cooking and at the table instead of salt.
- Cook rice, pasta, and hot cereals without salt. Cut back on instant or flavored rice, pasta, and cereal mixes, which usually have added salt.
- Select low-salt versions of canned meats such as tuna.
- Remove the saltshaker from the dining table.
- Choose "convenience" foods that are low in sodium. Cut back on frozen dinners, mixed dishes like pizza, packaged mixes, canned soups or broths, and salad dressings, all of which often have a lot of sodium.
- When available, buy low- or reduced-sodium or no-salt-added versions of such foods as:

> canned soup, dried soup mixes, bouillon
> canned vegetables and vegetable juices

cheeses, lower in fat
margarine
condiments such as ketchup and soy sauce
crackers and baked goods
processed lean meats
snack foods, such as chips, pretzels, and nuts

- Learn ways to cook that keep down the sodium in your diet.

Salt adds flavor to food and heightens existing flavors. The more salt that is added to our diets, the more we crave the intense flavors it creates. Unfortunately, as we've seen, the results of this are harmful to our bodies. It's important for most of us to try to cut down on salt, because reducing the sodium in our diets is key to keeping our blood pressure at a healthy level.

Keep in mind that after reducing the salt in your diet, you may initially find that food tastes bland. Soon enough, though, you will become reaccustomed to how food tastes in its natural form. You may even find that many of the processed foods you used to eat taste much too salty.

Following our low-salt version of the DASH diet requires a greater commitment on your part than the original diet. However, in keeping with the DASH philosophy, a DASH diet that is reduced in salt isn't a diet of deprivation or one that's too complex or inconvenient to follow. You are not prohibited from eating favorite foods, including nuts, cookies, and meat. As with the original DASH diet, all foods in the low-salt version can be found on grocery store shelves and require no special preparation. In time your taste buds will adjust to this healthier way of eating, and soon you'll develop a preference for foods in their natural, low-salt state.

5

────────────⋁────────────

DASH Plus:
Weight Loss, Exercise, and Limiting Alcohol Consumption

In the previous chapter we showed you how to optimize the DASH diet by reducing salt. In this chapter we will show you the three other effective ways to further enhance the effectiveness of the DASH diet:

- Get your body fat to a healthy level.
- Start an exercise program.
- Limit your alcohol consumption.

Bring Your Body Fat to a Healthy Level

About half of all Americans are overweight. A more accurate term, though, is *overfat*. That's because muscle weighs more than fat. Some heavily muscled people who register as overweight on height/weight tables may in fact be healthy and not too fat at all. But most of us who are overweight are carrying around too much fat. Being overfat makes you up to six times more likely to have high blood pressure. The term *obesity*, which also refers to body fat content, applies to a more extreme condition than overweight.

You can lower your blood pressure by losing body fat. Even a loss of only a few pounds of body fat can make a big difference in improving your blood pressure health. If you are over-fat and have a family history of hypertension, losing weight will reduce the chance you will develop high blood pressure.

Are You Overweight?

Healthy weight is best determined by working out your body mass index (BMI). BMI compares how much you weigh to how tall you are. A BMI of 25 is considered overweight, and 30 or above is obese. Calculate your BMI using the accompanying table on pages 48-49.

If Your BMI Is . . .	*You Are Considered . . .*
less than 20	underweight
20–24.9	normal/healthy weight
25–30	overweight
more than 30	obese

Getting Older, Getting Heavier?

It is especially important to be vigilant about fat gain in middle age. The weight gain we experience as we get older is fat. Don't ignore modest weight gains of 5 to 10 pounds. Although these initial gains in fat may not themselves cause high blood pressure, they can represent the beginning of a long-term increase in body fat that may eventually contribute to hypertension. It becomes a lot more difficult to lose the fat gain when it gets to 30 or 40 pounds.

Using the DASH Diet to Lose Weight

You can lose weight on any type of diet. All you need to do is eat fewer calories than your body needs. Easy to say, hard to do. But the DASH diet, with its emphasis on fruits and vegetables and low-fat foods, is ideally suited for weight loss. Adapting the DASH diet so it meets the needs of the person trying to lose weight is the focus of the next chapter.

Start an Exercise Program

Exercise can also lower your blood pressure. Scientists believe this happens because when you're exercising and the blood is pumping through your body faster than normal, this process clears the arteries and makes them more elastic, thereby reducing the amount of pressure against the artery walls.

In addition to improving blood pressure health, exercise promotes fat loss, another important way to lower blood pressure (see page 45). Of course, exercising is good for you in many other ways.

Remember to consult your doctor before beginning an exercise program if any of the following applies to you:

- You have heart trouble or chest pain, or you have had a heart attack.
- You take medicine for high blood pressure.
- You are over 50 years old and do not exercise.
- You have a family history of heart disease at a young age.

The Benefits of Regular Physical Activity

Regular physical activity improves health in the following ways:

Hypertension-Specific

- Reduces the risk of developing high blood pressure.
- Helps reduce blood pressure in people who already have high blood pressure.
- Helps control weight.

What's Your BMI?

Find your height in inches in the left column. Look across that row to find your weight (in pounds). Your BMI is indicated at the top of that column.

BMI	19	20	21	22	23	24	25	26	27	28
Inches										
58	91	95	100	105	110	115	119	124	129	134
59	94	99	104	109	114	119	124	128	133	138
60	97	102	107	112	118	123	128	133	138	143
61	100	106	111	116	121	127	132	137	143	148
62	104	109	115	120	125	131	136	142	147	153
63	107	113	118	124	130	135	141	146	152	158
64	110	116	122	128	134	140	145	151	157	163
65	114	120	126	132	138	144	150	156	162	168
66	117	124	130	136	142	148	155	161	167	173
67	121	127	134	140	147	153	159	166	172	178
68	125	131	138	144	151	158	164	171	177	184
69	128	135	142	149	155	162	169	176	182	189
70	132	139	146	153	160	167	174	181	188	195
71	136	143	150	157	165	172	179	186	193	200
72	140	147	155	162	169	177	184	191	199	206
73	144	151	159	166	174	182	189	197	204	212
74	148	155	163	171	179	187	194	202	210	218
75	152	160	168	176	184	192	200	208	216	224
76	156	164	172	180	189	197	205	213	221	230

Copyright 1999 George A. Bray

29	30	31	32	33	34	35	36	37	38	39	40
138	143	148	153	158	162	167	172	177	181	186	191
143	148	153	158	163	168	173	178	183	188	193	198
148	153	158	164	169	174	179	184	189	194	199	204
153	158	164	169	174	180	185	190	195	201	206	211
158	164	169	175	180	186	191	196	202	207	213	218
163	169	175	180	186	192	197	203	208	214	220	225
169	174	180	186	192	198	203	209	215	221	227	233
174	180	186	192	198	204	210	216	222	228	234	240
179	185	192	198	204	210	216	223	229	235	241	247
185	191	198	204	210	217	223	229	236	242	248	255
190	197	203	210	217	223	230	236	243	249	256	263
196	203	209	216	223	230	237	243	250	257	264	270
202	209	216	223	230	236	243	250	257	264	271	278
207	215	222	229	236	243	250	258	265	272	279	286
213	221	228	235	243	250	258	265	272	280	287	294
219	227	234	242	250	257	265	272	280	287	295	303
225	233	241	249	256	264	272	280	288	295	303	311
232	240	247	255	263	271	279	287	295	303	311	319
238	246	254	262	271	279	287	295	303	312	320	328

General

- Reduces the risk of dying prematurely.
- Reduces the risk of dying from heart disease.
- Reduces the risk of developing diabetes.
- Reduces the risk of developing colon cancer.
- Reduces feelings of depression and anxiety.
- Helps build and maintain healthy bones, muscles, and joints.
- Helps older adults become stronger and better able to move about without falling.
- Promotes psychological well-being.
- Increases energy level and lets you do more without becoming fatigued.

Is Moderation the Exercise Answer for You?

It isn't necessary to participate in strenuous exercise to improve your blood pressure health. The phrase "no pain, no gain" is outdated and erroneous. Recent studies have shown that regular, *moderate-intensity* exercise offers blood pressure benefits similar to those of vigorous physical activity. What is moderate? During moderate exercise you should not get so out of breath that you cannot carry on a conversation.

Moderate-intensity exercise is especially important for people who are elderly or obese and who might therefore not easily tolerate vigorous activities like jogging and aerobics. One of the great benefits of moderate exercise is that as you get into better shape, you will be able to do more—walk farther, faster, and for a longer time—and still be engaged in "moderate" exercise.

For most people with hypertension, a total of 30 minutes of moderate-intensity exercise at least five days a week (preferably every day) is enough to help start a downward trend in blood pressure. It isn't necessary to exercise for 30 minutes

Moderate-Level Physical Activities

Examples of moderate-level activities are as follows:

- Walking briskly (3–4 miles per hour)
- Home care and general cleaning
- Home repair, such as painting
- Mowing the lawn (with power mower)
- Gardening
- Dancing
- Table tennis/Ping-Pong
- Golf (walking the course)
- Fishing (standing and casting, walking, or wading)
- Swimming (at a moderate pace)
- Cycling (at a moderate speed of 10 miles per hour or less)
- Canoeing or rowing (at a speed of about 2–3.9 miles per hour)

Source: Adapted from Pate et al., *Journal of the American Medical Association* 273 (1995), page 404.

continuously—you can break up the time into 10-minute increments. An excellent form of moderate-intensity exercise is walking. If you haven't exercised for some time, walking may be the way to start getting in shape. Use the beginner's program in the accompanying table. If you start with ¼ mile and it's no strain, you can advance to ½ mile the next time out. If ¼ mile makes you a little tired, stick with that distance for two or three more outings, until your legs and lungs get stronger. Remember, you don't need to exhaust yourself or get out of breath to benefit from exercise.

A Walking Program to Fit Your Needs

Exercise has special benefits for people who have high blood pressure, and walking is a safe and effective way to exercise. Of the three different walking programs below, one should meet your needs. Remember not to overdo it early on and, if necessary, to get clearance from your doctor before you start.

Beginner's Program
(if you are elderly, obese, or very unfit)

WEEK	DISTANCE (miles)	DURATION (minutes)	FREQUENCY (times/week)
1	¼	10–15	2–3
2	½	12–15	2–3
3–4	¾–1	20–25	3
5–6	1–1½	20–30	3–4
7–8	1½–2	27–36	3–4
9–10	2–2½	35–44	4
11–12	2½–3	43–51	4
13–14	2½–3	40–48	4
15+	3–3½	48–56	4–5

Moderate-Intensity Program
(if you are reasonably "in shape")

WEEK	DISTANCE (miles)	DURATION (minutes)	FREQUENCY (times/week)
1	½–1	8–15	2–3
2	1½	23	2–3
3–4	1½–2	21–26	3
5–6	2–2½	29–39	3–4
7–8	2½–3	35–42	3–4
9–10	2½–3	34–41	3–4
11–12	2½–3	33–39	4
13–14	3–3½	39–46	4–5
15+	3½–4	46–52	4–5

**Advanced Program
(if you are regularly active)**

WEEK	DISTANCE (miles)	DURATION (minutes)	FREQUENCY (times/week)
1	½–1	6–12	2–3
2	1½	18	2–3
3–4	1½–2	18–24	3
5–6	2–2½	23–29	3–4
7–8	2½–3	28–33	3–4
9–10	3–3½	33–39	3–4
11–12	3–3½	32–37	4
13–14	3½–4	37–42	4–5
15+	3½–4	35–40	4–5

You should also try to work physical activity into your everyday life. For example, take the stairs instead of the elevator; park at the far end of the parking lot and walk to the office or store; mow the lawn and rake the leaves; and carry your groceries to the car and into the house.

It's amazing how small lifestyle changes can make a big difference to fitness. A recent Boston study showed that peple who take the subway to work are usually in significantly better shape than people who drive, because they tend to walk to the subway line and often stand during the ride.

Launching a Vigorous Exercise Program

The new information about exercise intensity—that it doesn't have to leave you exhausted—doesn't mean that if you were thinking about taking up racquetball again or training for a marathon, you should abandon your plans. High-intensity activity has its place, and certainly it can improve fitness, help control weight, make you feel good, and of course, lower your blood pressure. This kind of exercise program may not be for everyone, but it may be for you.

Remember, anyone with hypertension needs to consult a physician before beginning a vigorous exercise program.

Here are some tips to help you make exercise a habit:

- Choose an activity you enjoy.
- Tailor your program to your own fitness level.
- Set realistic goals.
- Choose an exercise that fits your lifestyle.
- Give your body a chance to adjust to your new routine.
- Don't become discouraged if you don't see immediate results.
- Don't give up if you miss a day; just get back on track the next day.
- Find a partner for a little motivation and socialization.
- Build some rest days into your exercise schedule.
- Listen to your body. If you have difficulty breathing or experience faintness or prolonged weakness during or after exercise, consult your physician.
- Try to do something every day—a little exercise is better than none at all.

Limit Your Alcohol Consumption

In the last few years much has been made of the potential "benefits" of drinking alcoholic beverages. Evidence does suggest that two alcoholic drinks a day for men and one for women is good for heart health.

Still, if you drink three or more drinks a day, you *increase* your risk of developing high blood pressure. Excessive alcohol consumption increases the flow of adrenaline, a hormone that constricts blood vessels, which in turn causes blood pressure to rise. Excessive alcohol consumption also reduces the effectiveness of blood pressure medication.

Smoking and Hypertension

Smoking cigarettes threatens your health in several important ways. Everyone thinks of the connection between smoking and lung disease, especially cancer. But smoking is also a very powerful cause of hardening of the arteries. It can temporarily increase your blood pressure because of the nicotine in each cigarette. But the bigger health concern is the long-term consequence of blood vessel damage.

If you smoke, quitting will reduce the harm to your blood vessels and overall health and will optimize the effectiveness of the DASH diet.

For more information on smoking cessation, seek information from these reputable medical organizations:

American Heart Association
7272 Greenville Avenue
Dallas, TX 75231
800-AHA-USA (242-8721)

American Cancer Society
1599 Clifton Road NE
Atlanta, GA 30329
404-320-3333

American Lung Association
1740 Broadway, 14th Floor
New York, NY 10019
212-315-8700

National Cancer Institute
Bethesda, MD 20894
800-4-CANCER (422-6237)

For pregnant women:
American College of Obstetricians and Gynecologists
409 12th Street SW
Washington, DC 20024
202-638-5577

Drinking too much alcohol contributes to a host of other health problems, including motor vehicle accidents, diseases of the liver and pancreas, damage to the brain and heart, an increased risk of many cancers, and fetal alcohol syndrome. Alcohol is also high in calories and devoid of nutrients.

The key is moderation. Men who have high blood pressure should limit the amount of alcohol they drink to no more than two drinks a day, and hypertensive women should keep it down to one drink. This is what counts as a drink:

- 1–1½ ounces of 80-proof or 1 ounce of 100-proof whiskey
- 5 ounces of wine
- 12 ounces of beer (regular or light)

What we set out to prove in the DASH study was that, *by itself*, a whole-food diet rich in fruits, vegetables, and low-fat dairy products and low in total fat and saturated fat would lower blood pressure in people with hypertension and prevent it from developing in at-risk individuals. Our goal was to

Stress and Hypertension

The relationship between emotional stress and hypertension is controversial. It's true that stressful situations can temporarily raise blood pressure, but there is no conclusive evidence that stress reduction or meditation can "treat" hypertension. For that reason there is no basis to recommend stress management as a treatment for this disease. By all means, participate in stress reduction programs, such as meditation and yoga, if they make you feel better, but remember they should not be a substitute for recognized hypertension therapies.

test the DASH diet by itself. Using strict scientific methods, we proved that the DASH diet alone could significantly affect blood pressure.

We believe the DASH diet can be the cornerstone of any program to manage high blood pressure. But why limit your program? By heeding the advice on alcohol restriction, physical activity, and weight management in this chapter, you can optimize the DASH diet and pave your way to even healthier blood pressure and better all-around mental and physical well-being.

6

Want to Lose Weight?
DASH Has the Answer

The DASH study proved that people who eat a whole-food diet rich in fruits, vegetables, and low-fat dairy products experience a beneficial lowering of their blood pressure. When we conducted the DASH diet, we neutralized several factors known to contribute to healthy blood pressure. That way we could be sure it was the foods themselves that were the cause of any blood pressure benefits. The antihypertensive factors we neutralized included reduced salt intake, increased exercise, and restricted alcohol consumption.

We also neutralized weight loss. We weighed the study participants every day and adjusted their food intake to keep their weight the same for the entire testing period.

Such is the blood-pressure-lowering power of the DASH diet that we managed to significantly lower the study participants' blood pressure even after neutralizing all those well-established antihypertensive factors. The participants were asked not to increase their physical activity or change their alcohol consumption. Nor did they have to lose weight.

Not only did our diet substantially lower blood pressure, but it didn't leave the study participants hungry. The DASH diet is a hearty eating plan that allows those who follow it to consume plenty of food every day. Most weight-loss diets leave people complaining about being hungry and tired. The DASH study participants reported unchanged or improved quality of life, largely because they were getting plenty to eat. In the field of nutritional science, this is a very significant finding.

People who eat the DASH diet don't have to lose weight in order to lower their blood pressure. However, we recognize that many people reading this book may have an interest in losing weight. If you are one of them, you have plenty of company. At any one time, tens of millions of Americans are dieting and spending a combined $30 billion every year on weight-loss products. Despite this, studies show that overweight and obesity in America are on the rise. Experts estimate that approximately 25 percent of women and 19.5 percent of men are obese — compared to approximately 15 percent and 11 percent, respectively, in 1980.

How can America be diet-obsessed *and* getting fatter? The fact is that many people who go on diets do not lose weight. And most people who do lose weight gain it back quickly after they stop dieting. Fad diets and diet pills may help some people lose weight in the short term, but they are not a substitute for adopting healthy eating habits for the long term.

Fortunately, it is possible to adapt the DASH diet to lose weight as well as to lower high blood pressure. In this chapter we'll show you exactly how to do it. But first, some background information on weight loss.

Fundamentals of Weight Loss

An effective weight-loss plan that keeps the pounds off requires that you take a multifaceted approach that includes educating yourself about how weight loss occurs, setting reasonable goals, changing the way you eat, and getting enough exercise.

Learning How Weight Loss Occurs

The term *calorie* is just a word we use to describe an amount of fuel or energy. You need a certain amount of body fuel (or number of calories) to get through the day and night. The number of calories burned in a day is different for different people. On average, men burn more calories than women; tall people burn more than short people; and active individuals burn more than sedentary ones. We'll show you how to estimate your calorie needs in the next chapter. But for this example, let's say that someone—we'll call him Bob—burns 2,500 calories getting through the average day (this is about right for a moderately active 160-pound man). If the food Bob eats every day provides 2,500 calories and he burns 2,500 calories, his weight will stay constant—he won't lose or gain. But if he starts eating 3,000 calories a day, his body will store the extra 500 calories as fat. If he does this every day for a week, he'll store 3,500 calories (500 calories/day × 7 days). Since every pound of fat contains 3,500 calories, Bob will gain 1 pound of body weight (fat) during that one week.

It works the other way too. If Bob, while burning 2,500 calories a day, reduces his food intake to 2,000 calories a day, his body will get the extra calories it needs by "borrowing" some of his body fat. If he continues this 2,000-calorie intake for one week, he will lose 1 pound (−500 calories/day × 7 days = −3,500 calories, or 1 pound).

This is why you can lose weight on any kind of "diet." Bob would still lose 1 pound per week if his 2,000 calories per day were all ice cream or all celery. He could consume 2,000 calories as 1 quart of ice cream or 631 stalks of celery. But, of course, neither would be a very healthful diet in the long term.

It's important to mention that, theoretically at least, you can also lose weight *without* reducing your food intake! If Bob starts walking 5 miles every day, he'll burn 3,000 calories a day instead of 2,500 (about 100 calories per mile). If he still eats his 2,500 calories a day, he will need to burn 500 calories of body fat to meet his energy needs. As a result, he will lose 1 pound of fat per week.

Of course, reducing food intake *and* exercising more is the preferred combination for weight loss.

Setting Reasonable Weight Goals for Yourself

To lose weight safely, you need to determine a realistic weight goal. The graph on the following page offers a range of suggested weights for adults, based on height.

If you're still unsure what your weight goal should be, consult a physician, dietitian, or nutritionist, who can help you set a reasonable goal.

Part of setting a reasonable goal includes how fast you try to reach it. The healthiest and longest-lasting weight loss occurs when a person loses 1 or 2 pounds a week. A loss of 1 pound a week can be attained by eating 500 calories less than you usually do every day or by decreasing how much you eat every day by 250 calories and increasing how much you exercise by 250 calories.

Eating a Diet Based on Moderation, Variety, and Balance

The three pillars of a healthy diet are moderation, variety, and balance. Moderation refers to not eating too much or too little of any one food or nutrient. Variety means eating a range of items from the food groups emphasized in the DASH diet. Balance involves making sure that you eat appropriate quantities of each food group and especially that you don't eat too much from those food groups that should be eaten in limited amounts, especially fats and oils and sweets.

Are You Overweight?

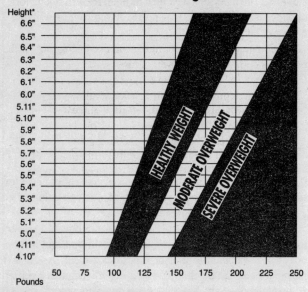

Heights are without shoes. Weights are without clothes. The higher weights apply to people with more muscle and bone, such as many men.

Source: U.S. Department of Agriculture, *Report of the Dietary Guidelines Advisory Committee on the Dietary Guidelines for Americans, 1995, to the Secretary of Health and Human Services and the Secretary of Agriculture,* pages 23–24.

Customizing the DASH Diet for Weight Loss

With all this as background, how can you use the DASH diet to lose weight?

To use the DASH diet for weight loss, calculate your calorie needs as the formula in chapter 7 suggests. Then *subtract 500 calories* from that and find the food servings that match your new, lower-calorie target. Don't worry if your calorie

Don't Believe the Hype

Fad weight-loss diets usually fall into one of several categories. Here are a few of those diets and what nutritional science thinks of them.

"Miracle Food" Diets

Certain diets promote one miracle food with special properties that will cause you to lose weight. Eating one food to the exclusion of all others may indeed result in weight loss—that's because eating just one food gets boring and usually you end up eating less of it! Furthermore, such diets discourage you from eating a balanced diet, the key to good nutritional health.

High-Protein/Low-Carbohydrate Diets

The theory behind these diets is that carbohydrates are "bad" because so many people are insulin-resistant and eating carbohydrates causes them to gain weight. Promoters of these diets point out that people who follow the high-carbohydrate diet that most qualified nutritionists recommend are fatter than they were before. What they neglect to tell you is that people are eating more calories, which is the *real* reason people are fatter.

High-Fiber/Low-Calorie Diets

Fiber is an important part of heart-healthy eating. A diet high in fiber can also help people trying to lose weight because fiber-rich foods are filling and low in calories (fiber cannot be digested). However, just because some is good doesn't mean a whole lot is better. Eating more than 50–60 grams of fiber a day can cause cramping, bloating, and diarrhea. Also, eating very high amounts of fiber doesn't necessarily guarantee weight loss. The only dietary modification that can do this for sure is eating fewer calories.   →

Liquid/Low-Calorie Diets

Over-the-counter liquid meal replacements and very-low-calorie diets should not be used for long-term weight loss, and they actually plateau after three months. Although they serve a short-term purpose, they do not foster good eating habits.

Fasting

Fasting has been recommended for years to purify the body or start a weight-loss program. Actually, fasting just deprives your body of nutrients. You end up with low energy, weakness, and lightheadedness—not weight loss. And when carbohydrates are not available for energy, substances called ketones can build up and stress the kidneys, which can be harmful to your health.

Be wary of claims that sound too good to be true. When it comes to weight-loss products and services, you should be particularly skeptical of claims containing words and phrases such as:

easy	magical	exotic
effortless	breakthrough	secret
guaranteed	new discovery	exclusive
miraculous	mysterious	ancient

target doesn't exactly match a calorie level in the servings table. Just pick the calorie level closest to your target. Remember, eating 500 calories a day less than you burn will lead to a loss of 1 pound of body fat per week. This is a good, safe rate of weight loss. You will have plenty of energy and will not feel totally food deprived. Very-calorie-restricted diets are difficult to adhere to. Besides, the DASH diet, which is rich in fruits and vegetables, contains a lot of nat-

---

Don't Forget About Exercise

Remember, there are two primary directives in weight loss—eat less and exercise more. Losing weight, as we explained, is simply a matter of using up more calories than you consume. To "use up" more calories, you need to be more active.

Chapter 5 contains detailed information about exercise, including a walking program for people with hypertension.

Important: If you exercise to lose weight, you will experience special blood pressure benefits. Exercise relaxes the arteries and thereby relieves blood pressure. Even if your blood pressure doesn't go down in response to exercise—which occasionally happens—studies show you are less likely to suffer severe medical problems if you are physically active than if you are sedentary.

---

ural fiber. This allows you to feel "full" without eating too many calories.

Because it is so well balanced, the DASH diet provides excellent overall nutrition as you lose those extra pounds.

The Substitution Solution

A diet that's "good for you" doesn't have to be dull or flavorless. There are plenty of high-quality, delicious food products available that will fit into your weight-loss program. Among the alternatives to regular-calorie, regular-fat foods are versions that are low-fat, no-fat, sugar-free, and low-calorie. New government labeling requirements make it easier to locate these products on store shelves (see page 69).

Modifying your diet with healthier substitutions is quite straightforward—you replace regular-fat and regular-calorie choices with foods and beverages that are lower in fat and calories, and you also alter your cooking methods. It's as simple as substituting nonfat or 1 percent milk for whole milk in your morning cereal, drinking diet soda instead of sugared soda at lunchtime, or enjoying steamed or boiled vegetables instead of fried or creamed vegetables at dinner. These simple substitutions will help bring meals in line with the DASH recommendations and will also help you reduce calories if you want to lose weight on the DASH diet.

The "substitution solution" is certain to influence your weekly preferences, then your monthly choices, and before long you will find yourself choosing healthier foods as a matter of habit. Meanwhile, here are some suggestions to get you started:

Instead of . . .	*Try . . .*
whole milk	nonfat dry milk, skim, or 1% milk
regular cheese	reduced-fat cheese
fried foods	baked, broiled, steamed, microwaved, or roasted meat, fish, poultry, and vegetables
oils, salad dressings, sour cream, mayonnaise	reduced-calorie or reduced-fat salad dressings and sour cream, low-fat or nonfat plain yogurt, mustard
butter, margarine	reduced-fat margarine, jam, jelly, preserves, low-calorie apple butter as a spread

ice cream	low-fat or nonfat frozen yogurt
rich desserts	angel food cake or sorbet
pudding	sugar-free pudding or gelatin
cake, pie, cookies, pastries	angel food cake, baked apple, fruit crisp, oatmeal cookies, ginger snaps, fresh or juice-packed canned fruit
doughnuts	bagels
snack crackers, chips	crisp breads, matzos, pretzels, rice cakes, melba toast, air-popped or microwaved popcorn

The Skinny on Fat

We all need some fat in our diets to maintain health. But compared to our ancestors, most Americans eat a diet that is too high in fat, especially saturated fats (those from animal products).

Saturated fats are the types of fat thought to be most responsible for fat-related health problems. The two other types of fat, monounsaturated and polyunsaturated, may have beneficial effects on health when consumed in moderation and as part of a healthy diet.

The DASH diet is low in total fat and saturated fat for two main reasons: to make room for foods rich in nutrients known to lower blood pressure and to lower cholesterol, which is a major risk factor for heart disease (a diet high in saturated fats causes cholesterol and other fatty substances to collect on the

---

Fat-Finding Mission

Saturated fats are solid at room temperature and come mostly from animal products, such as meat, lard, and butterfat (found in some cheeses, sour cream, heavy cream, and butter), as well as from coconut, palm, and palm kernel oils. Fats and oils that are liquid at room temperature are mostly unsaturated—either monounsaturated or polyunsaturated. Examples of monounsaturated fats are canola, olive, and peanut oils. Corn, soybean, and sunflower oils are high in polyunsaturated fats. Foods that contain mostly unsaturated fats include avocados, olives, and peanuts.

---

walls of your blood vessels). Although unsaturated fats may have health benefits, from the point of view of weight loss and weight control, they are *as high in calories* as saturated fats. Therefore, all fats need to be reduced in our diets to keep calories down.

When you're eating the DASH diet, only 27 percent of your diet is fat, compared to the average American diet, which is 34 percent fat. The DASH diet's 27 percent fat content is consistent with the American Heart Association's recommendations. Saturated fats account for only 6 percent of the DASH diet, while the average American diet is 16 percent saturated fat. The fats in the DASH diet come from meats, dairy, and grains, as well as from fats added to meals in the form of salad dressings, margarine or butter, and jellies and jams.

These are some ways you can trim some fat from your diet:

- Select lean cuts of meat, such as loin and round cuts, and trim all visible fat.
- Buy lower-fat versions of your favorite dairy products, such as skim milk and skim-milk-based cheeses.

- For added flavor, use herbs and spices in place of high-fat flavorings or sauces on vegetables, meats, poultry, and fish.
- Chill soups and stews and skim off the fat that collects on the surface.
- Choose low-fat or nonfat versions of your favorite salad dressings, mayonnaise, yogurt, and sour cream.
- Use low-fat or fat-free marinades to tenderize and add flavor to leaner cuts of meat.
- Use polyunsaturated or monounsaturated oil whenever a recipe calls for melted shortening or butter.
- Use vegetable-oil margarine in place of butter or lard. Look for whipped lower-fat tub margarine.

Remember, food labels can tell you more about the foods you eat and help you make the choices necessary to lower the fat in your overall diet. Learn how to read the Nutrition Facts panel on most packaged foods and what such claims as "low-fat" and "no-fat" mean.

Nutrition Facts Panel and Food Labeling

The Nutrition Facts panel is the rectanglar box of information found on food packaging. By law, most food labels must display a Nutrition Facts panel to help consumers make healthy food choices. Studies have shown that people who refer to the Nutrition Facts panel tend to be less overfat than those who do not.

What about using the Nutrition Facts panel specifically for weight loss? This is primarily a matter of paying attention to fat and calorie content. Fat is certainly not the only source of calories in food, but in the modern diet, fat is the densest source of calories. Be sure that the product is also low in calories. Many "low-fat" products contain plenty of calories in the form of sugars and other carbohydrates.

The Nutrition Facts panel makes it simple to identify foods high and low in fat. When you refer to the column of numbers that runs down the right side of a Nutrition Facts panel—known as % Daily Values—you will see that there is always a % Daily Values number for fat. When the %DV is less than 5 percent, the food item is considered low in fat, and when it is higher than 20 percent, the food is considered high in fat.

Where it comes to determining which foods should be part of a weight-loss diet, the Nutrition Facts panel is a much simpler resource than the confusing claims on the front of the packaging, even though the government's Food and Drug Administration now has very specific rules about what food makers can put on their labels to entice customers.

	% Daily Value*
Total Fat 12g	18%
Saturated Fat 3g	15%
Cholesterol 30mg	10%
Sodium 470mg	20%

Shedding Light on "Light"

"Light" (or "lite"), without any additional clarification, may be used only to describe a food that is significantly lower in fat, calories, or sodium compared to what the FDA calls a "reference food" (for example, regular potato chips would be the reference food for a light potato chip).

If a product is described as light, with no further explanation, you can be assured that only 25 percent of its calories are from fat.

Other Label Claims

Two other terms that play an important role in how health-conscious consumers choose foods are "reduced" and "less." Either claim may be used if a food contains at least a 25 percent reduction of the given nutrient when compared to the reference food.

The FDA has established "reference amounts" for 139 different food product categories. These represent the amount of a given food customarily eaten during a sitting.

Other labeling terms defined in the regulations include the following:

- *Fat-free:* Less than 0.5 gram of total fat for a given reference amount.
- *Calorie-free:* Less than 5 calories for a given reference amount.
- *% Fat-free:* Products that are labeled as being a certain percentage fat free must contain 3 grams or less of total fat for a given reference amount. A "100% fat-free" claim may be made only on foods that meet the criteria for "fat-free" and also contain less than 0.5 gram of fat per 100 grams and contain no added fat.
- *Cholesterol-free:* Less than 2 milligrams of cholesterol for a given reference amount and 2 grams or less of saturated fat for a given reference amount.
- *Saturated fat-free:* Less than 0.5 gram saturated fat for a given reference amount and no more than 0.5 gram of trans fatty acids.
- *Low-fat:* 3 grams or less of total fat for a given reference amount.
- *Low-calorie:* No more than 40 calories for a given reference amount (except sugar substitutes).
- *Low-saturated-fat:* 1 gram or less of saturated fat for a given reference amount and not more than 15 percent of calories from saturated fat.

Remember, though, that while it is helpful to know what these terms mean, they were created by marketing experts, not nutritionists. The easiest way to tell whether a food product is high or low in calories or a particular nutrient is to refer to the Nutrition Facts panel on the packaging.

Keeping It Off

For your weight-loss program to be considered a success, you have to keep the weight off in the long term. Many experts believe this is more difficult than losing the weight in the first place. Less than one-third of the people who lose weight are able to keep it off. Long-term weight-loss success depends on maintaining the good eating habits you developed while losing weight and also continuing the exercise program you began.

It takes time to make these new habits an ongoing part of your life. These are some ways you can continue to sustain your weight loss:

- Accept the fact that you will still be tempted by "fattening" foods.
- Realize you can eat tempting foods in moderation.
- Make the most of the low-calorie and low-fat choices available in your supermarket.
- Try new forms of exercise (by making exercise fun, you will likely stick to it).

It's important you get to know your eating habits — especially your bad habits. For example, do you overindulge when eating your favorite foods? Do you eat when you're stressed out or depressed? Do you use food as a reward? Keeping a food diary will help you identify bad habits and cut down on how much you eat.

Never let a temporary setback get you down or make you want to quit. Go right back to your winning ways!

Stay motivated and focus on your goals. Seek help if you cannot do it alone. Join a weight-loss organization or a health club. Your local hospital may even offer a weight-loss clinic. Also ask friends and family for support.

The basic principle behind weight loss—that you need to eat fewer calories than you use—is easy to understand but not necessarily easy to make a part of your life. When you have realistic goals in place and make a commitment to losing weight gradually by combining exercise with a modified version of the DASH diet, your chances of long-term success will be greatly enhanced.

PART THREE

DASH in Action

7

Putting DASH into Action:
How to Start Eating the DASH Way

Now it's time to put principles into practice and set DASH in action. In the next chapter we will provide you with expertly designed menu plans. But first we're going to teach you how to use the fundamentals of the DASH diet to create your own DASH eating system.

DASH in Three Easy Moves

Learning how to put DASH in action can be as easy as one, two, three.

1. Calculate your "calorie target" (how many calories you need to eat per day).
2. Find the DASH diet appropriate for your calorie target and learn the number of servings from each food group you should eat every day.
3. Learn what counts as a serving.

Step 1. Calculate your calorie target.

People have very different energy needs. A 180-pound active college student has different energy needs from, say, a 100-pound senior citizen who is wheelchair bound.

One of the first steps you need to take when putting DASH into action is calculating how many calories you should be getting every day. Once you've done this, it is easy to determine which version of the DASH diet you should be eating. Use the accompanying table to find out how many calories you need every day.

How Many Calories You Need Each Day

	Women		
Weight (pounds)	Less Active	Moderately Active	Very Active
100	1,178	1,473	1,669
110	1,296	1,620	1,836
120	1,414	1,767	2,003
130	1,532	1,915	2,170
140	1,649	2,062	2,337
150	1,767	2,209	2,504
160	1,885	2,356	2,671
170	2,003	2,504	2,837
180	2,121	2,651	3,004
190	2,239	2,798	3,171
200	2,356	2,945	3,338
210	2,474	3,093	3,505
220	2,592	3,240	3,672
230	2,710	3,387	3,839
240	2,828	3,535	4,006
250	2,945	3,682	4,173

Men

Weight (pounds)	Less Active	Moderately Active	Very Active
120	1,571	1,964	2,225
130	1,702	2,127	2,411
140	1,833	2,291	2,596
150	1,964	2,455	2,782
160	2,095	2,618	2,967
170	2,225	2,782	3,153
180	2,356	2,945	3,338
190	2,487	3,109	3,524
200	2,618	3,273	3,709
210	2,749	3,436	3,895
220	2,880	3,600	4,080
230	3,011	3,764	4,265
240	3,142	3,927	4,451
250	3,273	4,091	4,636
260	3,404	4,255	4,822
270	3,535	4,418	5,007

A *less active* person may do office work or typical household chores, but no specific exercise.

A *moderately active* person may participate in three to four sessions of aerobic exercise per week, lasting more than 20 minutes each. (Examples include brisk walking, jogging, bike riding, and recreational-level sports.)

A *very active* person may participate in five to seven aerobic sessions per week.

Those needing more than 3,000 calories could add one serving of grain, fruit, or vegetable and half a serving of dairy or meat for every increment of 500 calories.

If you are still unsure how many calories to eat every day, ask a registered dietitian or nutritionist for guidance or see Appendix B.

Step 2. Find the DASH diet appropriate for your "calorie target" and learn the number of servings from each food group you should eat every day.

Now that you know what your calorie intake should be, refer to the accompanying table, which tells you how many servings to eat every day from each of the food groups.

How Many Servings You Need Each Day from Each Food Group

	Grains	Vegetables	Fruits	Dairy foods
Calorie-Intake Range				
1,400–1,800	6	4	4	2
1,800–2,200	7	4	4	2½
2,200–2,600	9	5	5	3
2,600–3,000	11	6	6	3½

	Meats, poultry, and fish	Nuts, seeds, and legumes	Added fats and oils	Sweets
Calorie-Intake Range				
1,400–1,800	1½	¼	1	½
1,800–2,200	1½	½	2	½
2,200–2,600	2	½	3	1
2,600–3,000	2½	½	4	2

Serving suggestions are for the middle of the calorie-intake ranges. If you are in the lower end of a particular range, choose fewer numbers of servings from the added fats, sweets, and meat food groups. If you are in the higher end of the range, increase the number of servings you eat of vegetables, fruits, low-fat dairy products, and whole grains and whole-grain products.

Step 3. Learn what counts as a serving.

Examples of serving sizes are given in the table below. If you eat more than the stated amount, count it as more than one serving. If you eat less than 1 cup, count it as less than one serving. Although serving sizes don't have to be exact, try as far as possible to stay close to what counts as a serving size.

Food Group	*Serving Size*
Grains and grain products	1 slice bread ½ cup dry cereal ½ cup cooked rice
Vegetables	1 cup raw leafy vegetable ½ cup cooked vegetable 6 ounces vegetable juice
Fruits	6 ounces fruit juice 1 medium fruit ¼ cup dried fruit ½ cup fresh, frozen, or canned fruit
Low-fat or nonfat dairy foods	8 ounces milk 1 cup yogurt 1½ ounces cheese
Meats, poultry, fish	3 ounces cooked meats, poultry, or fish
Nuts, seeds, and legumes	1½ ounces or ⅓ cup nuts 2 tablespoons seeds ½ cup cooked legumes

Food Group	Serving Size
Fats and oils	1 teaspoon regular soft margarine, butter, or regular mayonnaise
	1 tablespoon low-fat mayonnaise or regular salad dressing
	2 tablespoons light salad dressing
Sweets	1 tablespoon maple syrup
	1 tablespoon sugar
	1 tablespoon jelly or jam
	½ cup Jell-O
	½ ounce jelly beans
	8 ounces sugared lemonade or fruit punch
	3 pieces hard candy
	½ cup sherbet
	1 Popsicle
	½ cup low-fat or nonfat frozen yogurt

Preparing to DASH

The following are important steps to take when getting ready to start eating the DASH way.

- Talk to your doctor about your plan and have him or her check your blood pressure.
- Set a firm date when you're going to start and mark it on your calendar. Don't go overboard on your eating in the meantime.
- Tell family, friends, and colleagues that you are going to start, and when. Ask them for support and understanding. If possible, get them to join you!
- As far as possible, get rid of non-DASH-friendly foods in your home, especially snacks such as high-fat ice cream, candy bars, and chips.
- Make a shopping list based on the meals you're planning to make and go to the supermarket to shop for the ingredients.
- Start changing your habits. Avoid eating in front of the TV or walking past a fast-food outlet where you often stop.
- Examine your past attempts to change your diet. Think about what worked and what didn't.

Vegetables

Can you imagine Italian food without tomato sauce? Or Mexican food without beans and salsa? How about Chinese food without onions and broccoli? Vegetables add taste, color, and texture to many of our favorite meals, and it's almost impossible to consider life without them. Rich in nutrients such as potassium, magnesium, and fiber and naturally low in calories, fat, and sodium, veggies are a key ingredient in the DASH diet.

The DASH diet contains more vegetables than the average American diet. Refer to the accompanying table for how many servings of vegetables to eat every day, based on your total calorie intake. Unsure which calorie level is for you? See pages 78–79.

How Many Servings of Vegetables You Should Eat Every Day

If you need:

> 1,800–2,200 calories a day—eat 4 servings
> 2,200–2,600 calories a day—eat 5 servings
> 2,600–3,000 calories a day—eat 6 servings

One serving equals:

> 1 cup *raw* leafy vegetable (e.g., spinach or lettuce—romaine, loose-leaf, Bibb)
> ½ cup *cooked* vegetable (e.g., spinach, kale, broccoli, cauliflower)
> ¾ cup vegetable juice (6 ounces)
> ½ medium-size potato or ¼ cup mashed potato
> ½ cup tomato sauce

Why don't Americans get enough veggies in their diet? Some people think they don't have time in their day to eat enough vegetables. Or that they don't taste good. But there are plenty of easy ways to prepare delicious vegetables that as part of the DASH diet can help you lower your blood pressure.

Selection Suggestions

In choosing what vegetables to buy and eat, the watchword is *variety*. About half your vegetable intake should be leafy greens and tomato-based products. The other half should be made up of a selection of veggies like green beans, peas, lima beans, peppers, potatoes, cucumbers, zucchini, eggplant, cabbage, broccoli, cauliflower, winter squash, sweet potatoes, and onions.

Preparation Pointers

It doesn't matter whether you microwave, boil, or bake them — vegetables retain 80 percent of their nutrients during the cooking process. In general, though, you should cook vegetables only until "crisp-tender" in just enough water to create steam,

---

Starch Smarts

Starchy vegetables, such as potatoes, corn, green peas, and dried beans, are higher in calories than other types of vegetables. But calories really go up when starches are fried or when sweet or fatty sauces and seasonings are added, so avoid frying these vegetables to keep from adding fats and calories. Some other smart ideas for starches:

- Cook starchy vegetables in unsalted broth for added flavor.
- To retain the natural fiber in potatoes meant for mashing, don't peel them — scrub them and cook them with their "jackets" on.
- Instead of using sour cream, top baked potatoes with plain low-fat yogurt seasoned with herbs or low-fat cottage cheese whipped with a little lemon juice in a blender.
- Make your own homemade potato chips by thinly slicing Yukon Gold potatoes and baking them in the oven. Spraying them with nonstick cooking spray works well.

but not so little you burn the cooking container. When cooking on the stovetop, use only a small amount of water and keep a tight-fitting lid on the pot so the vegetables cook quickly. Cooking vegetables a long time can "cook out" nutrients, flavor, and bright colors.

These are two more vegetable preparation hints:

- Add less butter, margarine, salad dressing, honey, salt, and soy sauce to vegetables to keep down the extra calories, fat, sugars, and sodium. Instead, add herbs and spices to enhance flavor. Start with ⅛ teaspoon for four servings and then let your taste be your guide. Add pizzazz to steamed veggies with a squirt of lemon.
- Make your own salad dressings and dips. Creamy dressings and dips can be made with plain low-fat yogurt instead of sour cream or mayonnaise.

Refer to pages 113–121 for general guidelines on cutting down on fat, salt, and sugar when you're cooking at home.

Fruits/Fruit Juices

How many foods can you think of that are blue? There aren't many—unless you count fruits. This is testament to the extraordinary variety within this food group. Fruit can be crunchy or soft, sweet or tangy, huge or tiny, ready-to-eat or packed in a thick or spiky skin, and of course, beautiful or ugly (though some of the ugliest fruit tastes the best).

Fruits and fruit juices are an important part of the DASH diet because they are rich sources of fiber, minerals, and nutrients. They are also naturally low in calories, fat, and sodium, which, along with vegetables, makes them an ideal DASH food.

The DASH diet recommends you eat considerably more fruit than average Americans get in their diet. But with all the

Easy Ways to Crank Up
Your Veggie and Fruit Intake

Fruits and vegetables are rich in key nutrients associated with healthy blood pressure. Yet most people with high blood pressure don't eat enough of them. The average American eats only about 3 servings of fruits and vegetables a day combined. Here are some tips on increasing your consumption of fruits and vegetables to meet your goal of 8 to 10 servings a day:

Start early. At breakfast time an 8-ounce glass of orange or grapefruit juice and banana slices, berries, or raisins on your cereal give you a delicious, mineral-rich, low-fat, high-fiber head start.

You can take it with you. Fruits and vegetables are portable and give you a quick boost of flavor and energy anytime. Pack an apple, an orange, or a bag of carrot sticks, raisins, or dried apricots in your glove compartment, purse, or briefcase.

Belly up to the bar. Find a good salad bar in your neighborhood and close to where you work for times when you don't feel like preparing something yourself. Learn to make appropriate selections. If your workplace has a canteen without a salad bar, get together with a few colleagues and ask your employer to install one. And make sure the salad bar items offer plenty of what you need — in particular, appropriate leafy green vegetables in place of iceberg lettuce, and low-fat salad dressings in place of full-fat ones.

See-food diet. Put fruits and vegetables where you can see them and within easy reach. Keep a bowl of fruit on the counter in the kitchen. Make sure fruits and vegetables are clearly visible when you open the refrigerator.

→

See-food diet (cont.) Cut up your favorite vegetables and store them in resealable plastic bags. You're more likely to eat what you see.

Stock up. Go shopping on the weekend and buy plenty of fresh, frozen, canned, and dried fruits and vegetables for you to eat through the week.

When you're all alone. Are you shooting for three vegetables with dinner? That much food preparation can be a challenge, especially if you're just cooking for yourself or if other household members aren't interested in eating the DASH diet. Some tips for getting in that "third" vegetable without a lot of extra trouble:

- Don't forget about salad.
- Keep family-size bags of frozen peas, beans, and carrots in your freezer so you can microwave a handful for yourself at dinnertime.
- Check out our vegetable recipes in chapter 10. Several of them are suitable for freezing and reheating. Make a big enough batch to freeze several individual servings to enjoy later—with almost no extra work!

Night moves. At the end of the day, the microwave is a quick, convenient way to prepare vegetables that preserves their nutrient contents. Pop a potato in the microwave at dinnertime and top it with your favorite salsa for a quick meal. Add microwaved broccoli and corn to your tasty tater and you've got a colorful, tasty, and nutritious meal. For dessert, top a scoop of low-fat frozen yogurt with fresh berries or sliced peaches.

choices available, it shouldn't be too difficult to meet the DASH diet's recommended daily number of servings of fruit. You can get fruit in your diet in so many ways because it comes fresh, frozen, canned, dried, and as 100 percent juice. Refer to the table below for how many servings of fruit to eat every day, based on your total calorie intake. Unsure which calorie level is for you? See pages 78–79.

How Many Servings of Fruit You Should Eat Every Day

If you need:

> 1,800–2,200 calories a day—eat 4 servings
> 2,200–2,600 calories a day—eat 5 servings
> 2,600–3,000 calories a day—eat 6 servings

One serving equals:

> 1 medium-size apple, banana, orange, peach, pear
> ½ grapefruit
> ¾ cup juice (6 ounces)
> ½ cup canned or frozen fruit
> ¼ cup dried fruit (apricots, cranberries, currants, dates, figs, peaches, prunes, raisins)

Selection Suggestions/Preparation Pointers

Mix it up. Try to get at least some fruit from each of the following groups in your diet over the course of the week: citrus fruits (orange, lemon, grapefruit), berries (strawberries, blueberries), temperate-climate fruits (pear, apple, peach), melons (cantaloupe, honeydew), tropical fruits (banana, pineapple), and fruit cocktail–type mixtures. Fresh, frozen, canned, and dried fruits are all good for you, but if you choose processed fruits, remember to avoid those that have added fat, sugar, or sodium.

Breakfast is a great place to emphasize fruit. A big (12-ounce) glass of juice and a banana on your cereal: you've just had 3 fruit servings!

Making Sure Juice Is Really Juice

Juices are a healthy and convenient way to get plenty of fruit in your diet. The words "100% fruit juice" on the label are key to making sure what you're getting is real juice nutrition. Beverages labeled fruit drink, fruit cocktail, or fruitade may contain added sugars that often replace fruit nutrition. These added sugars usually increase calories. Some of these drinks may contain no juice at all. The key is to check the label to get the product you're looking for.

There are so many choices when selecting fruits. Have you ever tried kiwifruit? How about mangoes? Experiment with trying new fruit. Every month, buy a variety of fruit you've never eaten before.

Meanwhile, here are some new ways to prepare familiar favorites:

- Serve fruit wedges with chunks of reduced-fat cheese.
- Jazz up coleslaw and chicken or tuna salad with apple chunks, pineapple, or raisins.
- Toss grapefruit and/or orange sections in a fresh crunchy salad of mixed greens—the sweet citrus and crisp lettuce are an incredible combination.
- Add raisins, banana slices, or blueberries to cereal.
- Keep things fresh and fun by combining fruits with different flavors and textures, like red grapes and pineapple chunks.
- For a snack at work, grab an apple or orange, or make a ready-to-eat bag of sweet cherries or grapes.
- Eat dried fruit instead of candy. For a quick, handy snack to go, try dried dates, figs, prunes, raisins, apricots, or other dried fruit varieties.

- Grill fruit skewers over medium-hot coals for a fun-to-eat and tasty barbecue treat.
- Make a quick smoothie in the blender by pureeing peaches and/or nectarines, a touch of your favorite fruit juice, crushed ice, and a light sprinkling of nutmeg.
- Make frozen fruit kabobs using pineapple chunks, bananas, grapes, and berries.
- For fruit salad in seconds, open a can of mandarin oranges and empty into a bowl. Add sliced banana, sliced apple, and some blueberries or raisins.
- Make juice cubes by pouring 100 percent fruit or vegetable juice into an ice cube tray and freezing.

Buying and Storing Fruit
When shopping:

- Look for fruits and vegetables that appear fresh, not bruised, shriveled, moldy, or slimy. Don't buy anything that smells bad.
- Ask the produce manager to help you choose a fruit you're unfamiliar with. Ask for a taste and for handling and storing information or for a recipe card.
- Most fruits and vegetables are not "stock-up" items. They should be used within a few days.
- Keep produce in the top of the cart, because putting heavy groceries on top of produce will bruise it. Some items that seem sturdy, such as cauliflower, are actually very delicate and bruise easily.

When you get your fruit home:

- Keep most of your produce in the crisper, where it will last longer because of the slightly higher humidity level. Keep all cut fruits and vegetables in the refrigerator.

- Wash produce just before you use it. Don't wash it when you put it away.
- To ripen unripe fruits, such as peaches, plums, and avocados, place them in a ripening bowl or a loosely closed brown paper bag, not a plastic bag. The natural ripening gases they give off will be held around them to help them continue to ripen. To speed up the process, place a ripe banana or apple in the bag with the unripe fruit. Some fruit, such as pineapple, will not ripen after it is picked.

Dairy Foods (Milk, Cheese, and Yogurt)

Dairy products have been an important part of our diet ever since people started keeping animals as livestock. As an example, when the early pilgrims traveled to Plymouth, Massachusetts, in the early 1600s, they brought cows with them. Dairy products are an important part of the DASH diet because they are rich sources of calcium and other nutrients. Keep in mind, though, that "whole" dairy products are high in fat, so always try to choose low-fat or nonfat versions to keep down your total daily fat consumption.

The DASH diet contains more dairy products than most Americans eat. However, it's not difficult to get enough dairy in your diet once you learn how. Refer to the accompanying table for how many servings of dairy products to eat every day, based on your total calorie intake. Unsure which calorie level is for you? See pages 78–79.

How Many Servings of Dairy Products You Should Eat Every Day

If you need:

1,800–2,200 calories a day—eat 2½ servings
2,200–2,600 calories a day—eat 3 servings
2,600–3,000 calories a day—eat 3½ servings

One serving equals:

- 1 cup (8 ounces) skim milk, 1% low-fat milk, 2% low-fat milk
- ⅓ cup nonfat dry milk powder
- 1 cup low-fat cottage cheese
- 3 tablespoons grated Parmesan cheese
- ¼ cup (1 ounce) shredded part-skim mozzarella cheese
- 1½ ounces low-fat or nonfat cheeses, including cheddar and ricotta
- 1 cup (8 ounces) low-fat or nonfat yogurt, fruit flavored or plain
- ½ cup (4 ounces) low-fat or nonfat frozen yogurt

How to Pump Up Your Dairy Intake

Most Americans don't get enough dairy products in their diets. To increase your consumption of dairy products—milk, yogurt, and cheese—start at breakfast.

At breakfast:

- Eat cereal with a serving or more of skim or 1% milk.
- Make oatmeal with skim or 1% milk instead of water.
- Spread low-fat or nonfat ricotta cheese and honey or fruit preserves on toast.
- Jazz up low-fat or nonfat yogurt with wheat germ, granola, or crunchy cereal.

At lunch:

- Eat a container of yogurt.
- Top sandwiches with a slice of low-fat or nonfat cheese.
- Finish lunch with a glass of ice-cold skim or 1% milk.
- Make soup with skim or 1% milk.

At snack time:

- Sip on hot cocoa made with skim or 1% milk instead of coffee or tea.
- Munch on fresh vegetables with a dip made from low-fat or nonfat yogurt.
- Nibble on popcorn sprinkled with Parmesan cheese.
- Try a smoothie made with low-fat or nonfat yogurt and your favorite fruit.
- Try a coffee drink like caffe latte made with skim or 1% milk.

At dinner:

- Make scalloped potatoes with skim or 1% milk and low-fat or nonfat cheese.
- Add low-fat or nonfat cheese to a casserole or meat loaf.
- Top vegetables with melted low-fat or nonfat cheese.

At dessert time:

- Make pudding with skim or 1% milk.
- Try low-fat or nonfat yogurt or low-fat or nonfat cottage cheese mixed with fresh fruit.
- Top apple pie with a slice of low-fat or nonfat cheese.

Selection Suggestions/Preparation Pointers

Try to avoid eating ice cream, whole milk, and regular cheeses, or eat just a little of those items at a time. Choose lower-fat or nonfat dairy products as often as possible. Remember, if you're not eating low-fat or nonfat dairy items, the calories add up faster than the calcium.

For milk:

- Instead of whole milk, use skim or low-fat milk in soups, puddings, baked products, or sauces for casseroles.
- Substitute evaporated skim milk in recipes calling for regular evaporated milk.
- Try undiluted evaporated milk as a substitute for cream.

For cheese and yogurt:

- Try lower-fat cheeses, such as part-skim ricotta or mozzarella, or low-fat processed cheeses.
- Use cheeses lower in sodium. Natural cheeses vary widely in sodium but generally contain less than processed cheeses, cheese foods, and cheese spreads. "Low-sodium" cheese is also available.
- Use plain low-fat yogurt or whipped cottage cheese as a substitute for sour cream in dips, salad dressings, or toppings for baked potatoes.
- Drain plain low-fat yogurt in a strainer lined with cheesecloth. Season the drained yogurt with herbs and use as a spread in place of cream cheese.
- Substitute plain low-fat yogurt for some of the salad dressing or mayonnaise in recipes.
- When cooking with cheese, you can usually reduce or omit the salt in recipes.

Refer to pages 113–121 for general guidelines on cutting down on fat, salt, and sugar when you're cooking at home.

Lactose Intolerant? You Can Still Enjoy Dairy Products!

Some people have trouble eating dairy products because they get an upset stomach—gas, stomach pains, or diarrhea. This

Milk Matters—but
What Kind Should You Drink?

Milk is an important part of the DASH diet. We recommend skim or low-fat milk for two reasons. First, the extra butterfat in whole milk (and cheese) is *saturated* fat, which increases cholesterol levels. Second, whole milk contains more calories per serving (see table below). For example, an 8-ounce serving of whole milk contains almost twice as many calories as skim milk, and all those extra calories are butterfat. We'd prefer you to drink the skim milk and eat an apple for about the same number of calories as you would get from the glass of whole milk alone! We also recommend low-fat yogurt and cheeses for the same reasons.

Milk product	Fat content (grams)	Calorie content
1 cup milk, skim	0.4	80
1 cup milk, ½% fat	1	90
1 cup milk, 1% fat	3	102
1 cup milk, 2% fat	5	120
1 cup milk, whole	8	150
1 cup milk, chocolate (2%)	5	179
1 cup milk, chocolate (whole)	9	250
½ cup evaporated milk (skim)	0.4	97
½ cup evaporated milk (whole)	10	126

condition, "lactose intolerance," is especially prevalent in people of East Asian, African, and Middle Eastern descent.

If you have trouble digesting dairy products, try taking lactase enzyme pills or drops with dairy foods to make them more digestible. Both items are available at drugstores and supermarkets, and a number of companies manufacture them. The most popular brand is Lactaid, but health-food stores and pharmacy chains often offer their own version. Typical tablets contain 3,000 lactase units, and the usual dose is one or two tablets taken before you consume dairy products. You might have to experiment to see how many tablets you need.

Here are some other tips for people who are lactose intolerant but still want to consume beneficial dairy products:

- Drink milk in servings of 1 cup or less along with meals or snacks. If you still get symptoms, try even smaller amounts more often throughout the day.
- Try natural aged or ripened cheeses, such as Swiss and cheddar. Not only do these cheeses contain little, if any, lactose, but they are an important source of calcium and other essential nutrients.
- Choose yogurts that carry the "live and active cultures" seal. These "friendly" cultures act like lactase by breaking down lactose in the digestive tract. If you're consuming sweet acidophilus milk, cultured buttermilk, or yogurt without active cultures, make servings small and accompany them with other foods or a meal.
- Small (½-cup) servings of ice cream or frozen yogurt often don't cause symptoms.
- Lactose-reduced and lactose-free milk and milk products are available in many grocery stores.

Despite the fact that some degree of lactose intolerance is pretty common in African-Americans and in older people, we had very few problems with lactose intolerance in our participants in the DASH study.

Your doctor, a registered dietitian, or other health-care provider can help you find ways to enjoy milk and milk products if you have difficulty digesting lactose.

Grains (Bread, Cereal, Rice, and Pasta)

Grains are the most important food crop in the world. Virtually every culture has its staple grain—couscous in Morocco, barley in eastern Europe, and rice in much of Asia (40,000 varieties of rice are grown around the world). The American diet is no stranger to grains. Most of us have a variety of grain products at home, from breakfast cereal to bread to spaghetti.

Grains are an integral part of the DASH diet because they are important sources of fiber, minerals, and vitamins. When you're eating the DASH diet, you eat more servings of grains every day than from any other food group. Refer to the table below for how many servings of grains to eat every day based on your total caloric intake. Unsure which calorie level is for you? See page 78–79.

How Many Servings of Grains You Should Eat Every Day

If you need:

    1,800–2,200 calories a day—eat 7 servings
    2,200–2,600 calories a day—eat 9 servings
    2,600–3,000 calories a day—eat 11 servings

One serving equals:

    1 slice bread, whole wheat or white
    ½ medium-size bagel
    ½ cup cold cereal, such as bran flakes or shredded wheat
    ½ cup cooked rice, pasta, or cereal (such as oatmeal)
    1 medium cornbread muffin
    2 graham crackers or 4 saltine crackers

Selection Suggestions

Almost all your intake of grains and grain products should come from bread, pasta, rice, and cereal, which are lower in fat and sugar, not from baked goods such as croissants, muffins, doughnuts, cookies, and other processed grain products.

As far as possible, try to choose whole-grain products because they are higher in fiber. These are ways to maximize the whole-grain content of specific foods:

Breakfast cereal: Look for "whole grain" on the package. Check the ingredients list for the word "whole" preceding these ingredients: oats, wheat, rice, corn, barley.

Bread: Even though a bread has "whole grain" on its labels, it doesn't have to be made from 100 percent whole grain. Check the ingredients label; whole-grain flour should be the first flour listed.

Rice and pasta: Brown rice is the only whole-grain rice. Whole-grain pasta was once rare in the United States but is becoming easier to find. If your grocery or supermarket doesn't stock whole-grain pasta, ask the manager to order a selection.

Preparation Pointers

- Go easy on fats and sugars when you add spreads, sauces, and toppings to grain products.
- Salt and oil are not necessary when cooking pasta, rice, and hot cereals.
- Salt can be reduced or omitted from pasta and rice casseroles that have other ingredients containing salt, such as cheese, canned soup, or canned vegetables.

Grain Expectations

Exploring the world of grains is a great way to add variety to your diet and increase your consumption of healthy grains. If you make your own bread (looking for a reason to dust off that automatic breadmaker you bought?), try experimenting with some of the grains listed below.

When dining out or perusing the shelves of your local specialty store, look for these grains:

Spelt, an ancient grain related to modern hybrid wheat, has a nutty flavor and is especially good in whole-grain bread and pasta.

Amaranth is actually an herb seed, not a cereal grain, and was cultivated as far back as A.D 700. It is loaded with protein, calcium, and iron.

Teff is a staple in Ethiopia used to make a flat bread called *injera.* It is the world's smallest cereal grain. Teff is high in iron, protein, trace minerals, and B vitamins. It is a good ingredient for quick breads.

Triticale, the world's first hybrid grain, is a combination of wheat and rye and has more protein than either. It is especially good in pilafs.

Job's tears (sometimes called Juno's tears) is an ancient grain originating in China. It has a natural sweetness and is delicious in soup, stuffing, or porridge.

Meat, Poultry, and Fish

Most Americans like to eat meat. Even many non-meat-eaters get a craving for meat when they smell bacon sizzling in a frying pan or a burger grilling on the barbecue. Meat, poultry, and fish are excellent sources of high-quality protein and important vitamins and minerals. However, 6 ounces a day of lean animal protein—about two servings—is all the meat, poultry, and fish you need to eat to be healthy. Any more than that and you are probably getting too much saturated fat in your diet. Meat, poultry, and fish should occupy a supporting role in a diet chiefly composed of fruits, vegetables, and whole grains.

The DASH diet recommends you eat less meat, poultry, and fish than the average American eats. Reducing the amount of meat you eat and making healthier meat-eating choices are easy, once you know how.

Another recommendation is that you try to achieve a balance between the three main forms of animal protein—meat, poultry, and fish. Americans tend to eat more red meat than poultry and fish. Yet poultry contains less saturated fat than meat, and most types of fish are lower in saturated fat than even poultry. Fish is especially underrepresented in the American diet, in part because we lack the knowledge of how to shop for and cook it. Yet fish is being increasingly recognized as a food that can be extremely beneficial for your health.

Refer to the accompanying table for how many servings of meat, poultry, or fish to eat every day, based on your total calorie intake. Unsure which calorie level is for you? See pages 78–79.

How Many Servings of Meat, Poultry, and Fish You Should Eat Every Day

If you need:

1,800–2,200 calories a day—eat 1½ servings
2,200–2,600 calories a day—eat 2 servings
2,600–3,000 calories a day—eat 2½ servings

One serving equals:

3 ounces cooked* lean meat, including beef, veal, and pork
3 ounces cooked* skinless white-meat poultry, including turkey and chicken
3 ounces cooked* fish and shellfish
1 ounce low-fat luncheon meats

*Note: A 3- to 4-ounce piece of cooked meat is about the size of a deck of cards.

Selection Suggestions

- All fish are naturally low in saturated fat, so choose fish instead of poultry or beef at least twice a week.
- When buying red meat, choose lean cuts. For beef, look for eye of round or top round. For veal, select ground veal or veal shoulder, cutlets, or sirloin. Pork lovers should go with lean tenderloin, sirloin, and top loin. Lamb lovers should try the leg or shank.
- Buy chicken and turkey without skin or remove the skin before cooking. White meat contains less saturated fat

---

What's All This About Fish and Omega-3 Fatty Acids?

Aside from its role in the DASH diet as an important source of healthy animal protein, fish offers another important reason to make it a part of your diet. Increasing scientific evidence is showing that foods such as fish that are rich in omega-3 fatty acids are good for your heart.

Omega-3 fatty acids help lower the fat in your blood known as triglycerides, reduce the tendency for dangerous clots to form in the blood, and reduce the risk of irregular heartbeat (arrhythmia) and even sudden death. A paper published in the *Journal of the American Medical Association* (January 1998) showed that consuming at least one meal of fish a week—compared to eating fish less than once a month—was associated with a 52 percent lower risk of heart attack.

A bonanza of omega-3 fatty acids is available in fatty fish such as salmon, anchovies, mackerel, albacore tuna, herring, and sardines packed in oil, but even lean cod, flounder, lobster, and crab provide this heart-healthy substance.

---

than dark meat. Try fresh ground turkey made from white meat, such as the breast.

- Limit goose and duck, which are high in saturated fat, even with the skin removed.

Preparation Pointers

- The rule of thumb for cooking fin fish, such as salmon, tuna, swordfish, cod, and haddock, is to bake it at 450°F for as little as 10 minutes per inch of thickness (always measure at the thickest point of the flesh), turning the fish halfway through the cooking time. Fish should be cooked until it is opaque in color and flakes easily when you touch it with a fork.
- Seafood is lower in fat, but avoid fried fish covered with a greasy batter or swimming in butter.
- Remove the skin from poultry. Taking the skin off a half breast of roasted chicken reduces the fat from 8 to 3 grams and the calories from about 195 to 140.
- Cut the fat off meat. Trimming the fat off a 3-ounce piece of broiled sirloin steak lowers the fat from 15 to 6 grams and the calories from 240 to 150.
- Broil, roast, or boil meat instead of frying it.
- Drain the fat after cooking ground beef.
- Cook with little or no oil, using nonstick pans.
- Place meat on a rack when roasting, broiling, or braising so the fat can drain away.
- Baste with unsalted broth, unsalted tomato juice, or fruit juice rather than with fatty drippings.
- If using ham or another cured meat in a recipe, omit the salt and avoid using other ingredients high in sodium.
- Go easy on commercially prepared products, such as barbecue sauce, which are often high in sugar and sodium or both.

- Use fewer high-sodium condiments, such as soy sauce and dill pickles.
- Steer clear of fatty processed meats, such as bologna, salami, hot dogs, sausages, and bacon, to avoid fat overload.
- Always follow proper safety practices for meat (see page 105).

Lowering Your Meat Intake

Often people eat a large portion of meat as a main course and don't get enough vegetables or grains. To help change your diet, try some of the following tips:

- If you currently eat large portions of meat, cut back by half or one-third at each meal.
- Prepare two or more vegetarian-style meals (meatless) every week.
- Include more servings of vegetables, rice, pasta, and beans so that you need less meat to make a satisfying meal. Casseroles, pasta dishes, and stir-fries often include less meat and more vegetables, grains, and beans.
- Purchase less meat. If it's not there, you won't eat it.

Refer to pages 113–121 for general guidelines on cutting down on fat, salt, and sugar when you're cooking at home.

Food Safety Basics

Wash hands and surfaces often:

- Always wash your hands with soap and warm running water before handling food.
- Always wash cutting boards, knives, utensils, dishes, and countertops used to cut meat with soapy hot water right away—before you put other foods in contact with them.
- Consider using paper towels to clean up kitchen surfaces. If you use cloth towels, dishcloths, or sponges, wash them often, and especially each time they touch raw meat, poultry, or seafood juices. Use hot soapy water or the hot-water cycle of the washing machine.

Don't cross-contaminate:

- Store raw meat, chicken, turkey, and seafood in a sealed container in the refrigerator.
- Keep raw meat, chicken, turkey, and seafood away from foods that will not be cooked and foods that are already cooked.
- Never place cooked food on a plate or cutting board that previously held raw meat, chicken, turkey, or seafood.

Cook to proper temperatures:

- Use a food thermometer to make sure meats, chicken, turkey, fish, and casseroles are cooked to a safe internal temperature.
- Cook roasts and steaks to at least 145°F.
- Cook ground meat to at least 160°F.
- Cook whole chicken or turkey to 180°F.
- Cook eggs until the yolk and white are firm, not runny. Don't use recipes in which eggs remain raw or only partially cooked.
- Cook fish until it flakes easily with a fork.   →

Refrigerate promptly:

- Thaw frozen foods in the refrigerator, not on the kitchen counter. You can also thaw foods under cold water, changing the water every 30 minutes. Or use a microwave oven.
- Refrigerate or freeze leftover foods right away. Meat, chicken, turkey, seafood, and egg dishes should not sit out at room temperature for more than 2 hours.
- Divide large amounts of leftovers into small, shallow containers for quick cooling in the refrigerator.
- Keep your refrigerator at 40°F or below. Don't pack the refrigerator. Cool air needs to circulate to keep food safe.

Nuts, Seeds, and Legumes

Throughout history nuts, seeds, and legumes have been an essential part of mankind's diet. And no wonder—these foods are concentrated sources of important nutrients that are essential to our health. You are probably familiar with legumes because they are the main ingredient in split pea and lentil soups. The beans that you eat in Mexican food are also legumes.

Nuts, seeds, and legumes are a big part of the DASH diet because they are rich sources of protein and many vitamins and minerals. While the portions we recommend are small, these foods are loaded with key nutrients. Maybe it is difficult for you to eat a half serving every day. If so, eat a whole serving every other day. But be sure to include these foods in your meal plans regularly.

The following are common examples of foods in this group:

Nuts: almonds, Brazil nuts, cashews, chestnuts, coconuts, hazelnuts (filberts), macadamia nuts, peanuts, pecans, pine nuts, pistachios, walnuts. You knew we'd find a food group for peanut butter, right?

Seeds: pumpkin, sesame, sunflower.

Legumes: soybeans (the most nutritious legume and the most common legume crop in the world), black-eyed peas, chickpeas (garbanzo beans), lentils, and black, red, white, navy, and kidney beans.

Keep in mind that nuts and seeds are also high in fat, so portions should be small. Refer to the accompanying table for how many servings of nuts, seeds, and legumes to eat every day, based on your total calorie intake. Unsure which calorie level is for you? See pages 78–79.

How to Get More Nuts, Seeds, and Legumes into Your Diet

Nuts

Nuts are an excellent snack food. In fact, if you kept a bowl of nuts on your coffee table or kitchen counter, you would find it difficult to resist consuming your daily requirement of half a serving! But because nuts are so high in fat, keeping a bowl or bag of nuts within reach may not be the wisest tactic—unless you have tremendous willpower. Consider these ways of getting enough nuts into your diet:

- Toss nuts into stir-fries, salads, and pasta dishes.
- Sprinkle nuts on top of frozen yogurt, ice cream, iced cakes, or iced cookies.
- Let nuts turn an ordinary recipe into something special. Sprinkle chopped nuts on top of a bowl of soup or your favorite casserole or vegetable.
- Start your day with nuts—experiment with different nuts in your favorite muffin or pancake recipe; sprinkle nuts on top of yogurt or oatmeal.

How Many Servings of Nuts, Seeds, and Legumes You Should Eat Every Day

If you need:

1,800–2,200 calories a day—eat 0.4 servings
2,200–2,600 calories a day—eat 0.5 servings
2,600–3,000 calories a day—eat 0.6 servings
Half a serving is probably appropriate for all groups.

One serving equals:

In general

⅓ cup or 1½ ounces nuts
2 tablespoons or 1½ ounces seeds
½ cup cooked dried beans/legumes

Specifically

⅓ cup almonds
½ cup cooked beans (dried), such as kidney, pinto, and navy
½ cup cooked chickpeas and lentils
⅓ cup cashews
⅓ cup mixed nuts
2 tablespoons peanut butter
⅓ cup peanuts
2 tablespoons sesame seeds
2 tablespoons sunflower seeds
3 ounces tofu, regular
⅓ cup walnuts

Seeds

Pumpkin seeds can be eaten raw or cooked in both sweet and savory dishes. They are delicious toasted and sprinkled, while hot, with low-sodium soy sauce, then tossed into a salad. Sesame seeds can also be added to main and side dishes, especially Asian ones, but are most often used as a decoration on cakes, candies, and other sweets. Sesame seed paste (tahini) is used in dishes such as hummus and some salad dressings. Sunflower seeds can be eaten whole, raw, or cooked. They can be added to breads and cakes or sprinkled over salads or breakfast cereals.

Legumes

Legumes are easy to prepare and versatile to use. They can be eaten alone, combined with other foods, or enjoyed as a snack. Because legumes pick up the flavors of the foods and spices they are cooked with, they are excellent "flavor sponges."

Legumes can be the main ingredient in a dish or liven up dishes like soups and casseroles. They can also be used as a meat replacer. Soy products such as tofu and texturized vegetable protein, which are available in most supermarkets, can be used in dishes like stir-fries and chili. Dried beans can also be used in place of meat in casseroles and soups. A classic vegetarian main course is a "meat" loaf made with nuts, seeds, and legumes, such as lentils or anoki beans. Many vegetarian cookbooks give a recipe for this loaf, which can be endlessly varied with different herbs and flavorings and different combinations of nuts and cereals. Chickpeas can be enjoyed as a roasted snack or used in salads and dips. Navy beans are the main ingredient in Boston baked beans.

Refer to pages 113–121 for general guidelines on cutting down on fat, salt, and sugar when you're cooking at home.

Added Fats and Oils

The fat in your diet is present not only in such foods as meat, dairy, grains, and nuts and in multi-ingredient recipes like pizza, but also in foods you add to other foods, such as salad dressing, margarine, and butter. To keep your fat intake at DASH diet levels, try to limit how much added fat gets into your diet. Refer to the accompanying table for how many servings of added fats and oils to eat every day, based on your total calorie intake. Unsure which calorie level is for you? See pages 78–79.

One note on the use of margarine. Margarine became popular as a substitute for butter when we learned that eating butterfat (a saturated fat) increases cholesterol levels. Although margarine is made from vegetable oils (unsaturated fats), the chemical process used to make it—hydrogenation—converts some of the oil to trans fatty acids, which can also increase cholesterol levels (although not as much as saturated fats). Hydrogenation makes margarine "hard" so it can hold a shape like butter. The harder the margarine, the more trans fatty acids it contains. Because of these concerns, we recommend using natural vegetable oils as much as possible. When you must use margarine, use the softer types, like tub margarine, because they contain less trans fatty acids.

Selection Suggestions/Preparation Pointers

- Use half the butter, margarine, or salad dressing you typically do now.
- Try low-fat or nonfat condiments, such as nonfat salad dressings, mayonnaise, yogurt, and sour cream.
- Use polyunsaturated or monounsaturated oil whenever a recipe calls for melted shortening or butter.

How Many Servings of Added Fats and Oils You Should Eat Every Day

If you need:

1,800–2,200 calories a day—eat no more than 2 servings
2,200–2,600 calories a day—eat no more than 3 servings
2,600–3,000 calories a day—eat no more than 4 servings

One serving equals:

1 teaspoon soft margarine or butter
1 teaspoon regular mayonnaise or 1 tablespoon low-fat
  mayonnaise
1 tablespoon salad dressing or 2 tablespoons light salad
  dressing
1 teaspoon oil (olive, corn, canola, safflower, or other
  vegetable oil)

- Use vegetable-oil margarine in place of butter or lard. Look for whipped, lower-fat tub margarine.
- When frying, stir-frying, or lining a baking pan, use vegetable-oil sprays to cut down on how much oil you use.

Refer to pages 113–121 for general guidelines on cutting down on fat, salt, and sugar when you're cooking at home.

Sweets

The DASH diet contains fewer sugary foods than the average American diet. To satisfy a desire for sweets, try diet fruit-flavored gelatin or, best of all, frozen, canned, or fresh fruit for dessert. Fruit gives you the sweetness you crave and lots of vitamins, minerals, and fiber. Refer to the accompanying table for how many servings of sweets to eat every day, based on your total calorie intake. Unsure which calorie level is for you? See pages 78–79.

How Many Servings of Sweets You Should Eat Every Day

If you need:

1,800–2,200 calories a day—eat no more than ½ serving
2,200–2,600 calories a day—eat no more than 1 serving
2,600–3,000 calories a day—eat no more than 2 servings

One serving equals:

1 tablespoon maple syrup
1 tablespoon sugar
1 tablespoon jelly or jam
½ cup Jell-O
½ ounce jelly beans
8 ounces sugared lemonade or fruit punch (8 fl. oz.)
3 pieces hard candy
½ cup sherbet
1 Popsicle
½ cup low-fat or nonfat frozen yogurt

Finding the Right Fruits for Desserts and Snacks

Many people enjoy snacks. Snacks can benefit your diet if you choose fruit or low-fat foods. Instead of chips, cookies, candy bars, or high-fat muffins, try some of the following:

- Fresh whole fruit or canned fruit packed in its own juice
- Dried fruit (easy to leave in the car or carry in a briefcase or purse)
- Unsalted pretzels or nuts mixed with raisins

- Graham crackers and other reduced-fat crackers
- Gelatin
- Low-fat and nonfat regular and frozen yogurt
- Popcorn, plain, with no added salt
- Raw vegetables, with nonfat ranch, blue cheese, or Thousand Island dressing as a dip

Many of the ideas in the section on "Fruits/Fruit Juices" (page 86) can be adapted for desserts and snacks that will satisfy a sweet tooth.

Healthy Hints for Home Cooking

The DASH diet recommends you try to limit fat, salt, and sugar in your diet. Here are some recommendations for how to do this when cooking at home using recipes.

To reduce the fat content of recipes:

When a recipe calls for . . .	*Instead use . . .*
whole milk	skim or nonfat milk nonfat dry milk, reconstituted
cream	evaporated skim milk
sour cream	plain nonfat yogurt for sour cream in food that is to be heated (mix in 1 tablespoon flour for each cup yogurt to prevent separation)

When a recipe calls for . . .	*Instead use . . .*
sour cream *(cont.)*	nonfat sour cream or plain nonfat yogurt with chopped green onions or chives as toppers for baked potatoes
full-fat cheese	low-fat cheese (part-skim mozzarella or reduced-fat cheese) combination of cheeses: for example, half Parmesan and half mozzarella to use on spaghetti low-fat or nonfat cottage or ricotta cheese for half or all the cheese called for in casseroles flavorful varieties in smaller amounts
mayonnaise	half the amount or less of imitation or light mayonnaise (light mayonnaise has half the fat content) plain nonfat yogurt or half nonfat yogurt and half light mayonnaise

oil, butter, or lard	vegetable margarine (soft stick or tub) or vegetable oil
	when sautéing, no more than 1–2 teaspoons oil, or use a nonstick pan or nonstick cooking spray
	water or low-sodium broth to cook vegetables
	microwave to cook vegetables without adding fat
	in baking, half the fat called for (for example, if recipe calls for ¼ cup oil, try 2 tablespoons or less), or use pureed fruit, such as applesauce
whole eggs	egg substitute, according to package directions (read label to make sure egg substitute does not contain cheese or other added saturated fats)
	2 egg whites for 1 egg
nuts	sparingly to add crunch to casseroles and baked products

When a recipe calls for . . .	*Instead use . . .*
nuts *(cont.)*	(no more than ¼ to ½ cup per recipe) *Note:* Nuts derive approximately 70–80% of their calories from fat.
creamed soups (chicken, mushroom, or celery)	½ can soup and ½ can skim milk homemade "cream" soup mix low-fat varieties
thickening with flour and butter	rapid boiling to reduce liquid cornstarch, rice or potato flour, or nonfat dry milk (no added fat) to thicken

To reduce the salt content of recipes:

When a recipe calls for . . .	*Instead use . . .*
salt	half the amount or less in recipes no salt (in some recipes—for example, muffins—salt can be completely

eliminated without
any change in
flavor)

fresh herbs: parsley,
thyme, basil, sage,
tarragon, mint, or
chives (use 3 times as
much chopped fresh
herbs as dried; dried
herbs and spices can
be freshened by
crushing them)

¼ teaspoon of a spice or
an herb, aromatic
bitters, or a shake-on
mix, such as
Mrs. Dash (*Note:*
There is no
connection between
the DASH diet and
the product
Mrs. Dash.)

dry mustard, ¼ teaspoon
at a time, to add
"kick" to meats,
vegetables, salads,
and grains

flavored vinegar in
soups, sauces, and
salad dressings or
over vegetables;
flavored vinegars
require less oil for
vinaigrette

When a recipe calls for . . .	Instead use . . .
salt (cont.)	1 teaspoon sherry added to clear broth
onion salt, garlic salt celery salt, or all-purpose seasoning	fresh onion or garlic onion or garlic powder celery seeds
canned broth or bouillon cube	fresh chicken or vegetable stock low-sodium bouillon cubes canned low-sodium broth
salted water	no salt in water *Instead for flavor, try adding:* garlic clove or piece of onion to water for cooking pasta 1 tablespoon vinegar to water for rice sprig of mint or small onion to water for boiling potatoes caraway, dill, or mustard seeds to water for cooking vegetables
canned tomatoes or canned tomato sauce	no-salt-added tomatoes or tomato sauce fresh tomatoes

tomato paste or tomato
puree (no-salt-added)
diluted with water or
stock to bring it up to
the right quantity

To reduce the sugar content of recipes:

When a recipe calls for . . .	Instead use . . .
sugar or honey	less sugar (for example, if recipe calls for ⅓ cup, try using ¼ cup or less) an extra ¼ teaspoon extract (vanilla, almond, or orange) in cakes or cookies to compensate for halved or reduced sugar fruit juice concentrate, such as apple juice (1 tablespoon equals 1 teaspoon sugar) unsweetened white grape juice (2 tablespoons equal 1 teaspoon sugar) when poaching fruit pureed fruit or dried fruit (dried fruits are high in calories, so use limited amounts)

When a recipe calls for . . .	*Instead use . . .*
sweetened to taste	dried fruit on cereals; for example, 2 level tablespoons of raisins, which contain 55 calories
	fresh fruit and juice concentrate stirred into plain nonfat yogurt
	fruit-flavored liqueur sprinkled over fresh fruit; also try NutraSweet sugar substitute over fruit
	grated orange or lemon rind in baked goods
	grated sweet vegetables, such as carrots, sweet potatoes, and parsnips, in casseroles that are too bitter
	cinnamon, ginger, nutmeg, or cardamom
	Note: Juices work best in sauces and cooked dishes. If you try them in baked goods, you must omit an equal volume of liquid from your

recipe to compensate
for the added liquid
volume of the juice.

packaged fruit-flavored
   gelatin

unflavored gelatin and
   fruit juices
packed gelatin
   sweetened with
   NutraSweet sugar
   substitute

DASH-Friendly Cooking Methods

Some methods of cooking are better for your health than others. Try some of the following methods if you are eating the DASH way.

Microwave: Microwaving cooks foods faster than most other methods. You don't need to add fat to meat, poultry, or fish, and you use little water for vegetables. Micro-cooking is an excellent way to retain the vitamins and color in vegetables. Follow the manufacturer's directions for best results.

Steam: Steaming is a good method for cooking vegetables without using fat. Try this method for both frozen and fresh vegetables, including asparagus, broccoli, carrots, spinach, and summer squash. Use a vegetable steamer or colander to hold the vegetables and place it in a pot with a little boiling water. Cover and cook the vegetables until they are just tender to preserve their color and vitamins.

Braise: Braising is used mainly for meats that need longer cooking times to become tender. Root vegetables are also good braised. Brown meat first in a small amount of oil or its own fat, then simmer in a covered pan with a little liquid. For the liquid, try using meat or poultry broth, cider, wine, or a combination of these for added flavor.

Barbecue: Roasting foods on a rack or a spit over coals is a fun, lower-fat way to prepare meat, poultry, fish, and even vegetables. Barbecuing gives a distinctive smoked flavor to any food. Trim the fat from meat to prevent a flare-up of flames and to reduce calories. If seasoning grilled food with a sauce, try one with less salt, sugar, and fat.

Broil: Broiling is a quick way of cooking foods under direct heat without added fat. It's great for poultry, fish, and tender cuts of meat. Use a broiling pan or rack set in a shallow pan to allow fat to drain away. If basting, use lemon juice, fruit juice, or broth for added flavor. Vegetables like onions, zucchini, and tomatoes can also be broiled.

Stir-fry: Quick and easy, stir-frying requires relatively little fat and preserves the crisp texture and bright color of vegetables. Heat a wok or heavy skillet, add just enough oil to lightly coat the bottom of the pan, add food, and stir constantly while cooking. Start with thin strips or diced portions of meat, poultry, or fish. When the meat is almost done, add small pieces of vegetables, such as broccoli, cauliflower, zucchini, sprouts, carrots, mushrooms, tomatoes, or green onions.

Roast or bake: Roasting takes somewhat longer than other methods but requires little work on your part. Poultry and tender cuts of meat may be roasted. Cook in the oven, uncovered, on a rack in a shallow roasting pan to drain the fat and allow the heat to circulate around the meat. Potatoes, sweet potatoes, winter squash, and onions can be baked. Simply wash, prick the skins, and place the vegetables on a baking sheet in the oven.

Boil or stew: Foods are cooked in hot liquids in these low-fat, low-salt methods. The liquid left after cooking can become a tasty broth or the base of a sauce; chill the liquid first and remove any fat that rises to the top. Starchy and root vegetables, such as potatoes, corn on the cob, lima beans, and turnips, are often boiled.

Simmer: Tough cuts of meat can be tenderized by simmering them in liquid for several hours. (A simmer is a slow boil

in which bubbles rise gently to the surface and barely break.) Add vegetables and herbs for an aromatic blend of flavors without salt.

Supermarket Savvy: How to Shop for DASH

We've spent the last several pages describing the different food groups and how to eat from these groups. Along the way we provided you with selection tips. Now let's look at how to put this knowledge to work in the grocery store.

Most grocery stores are laid out according to a fairly standard floor plan. As you enter the supermarket and follow the walls, you encounter the fresh fruits and vegetables first, then the meat section, the dairy department, and the breads and bakery. In the middle of the store is where you find packaged foods and impulse items that are often not on your shopping list. DASH-savvy shoppers know that shopping a grocery store's *perimeter* is the healthiest way to fill their grocery cart.

Produce Section

The produce section of the supermarket offers the widest variety of healthy fruits and vegetables, which are wonderfully nutritious food choices and part of the foundations of the DASH diet. They are excellent sources of vitamins, minerals, and fiber and are naturally low in calories, sugar, and fat. A few tips:

- Watch out for higher-fat foods like avocados, deep-fried nuts, and specialty dressings.
- Experiment with new or unusual fruits, vegetables, and spices.
- Buy packaged precut vegetables to make cooking faster and easier. Don't forget the salad bar: it's a quick stop for washed precut vegetables and fruit.

Meats, Poultry, and Seafood Section

The back of the store is usually where you'll find the meat, poultry, and seafood options. Remember to buy the freshest meat possible, as well as the leanest. If grams are not stated on a low-fat product, choose the one labeled "95% or less, fat-free."

Red Meats—Beef, Lamb, Pork, and Veal

Red meats include beef, lamb, pork, and veal. Use the following guide to find the leanest cuts of meat:

> Lean beef: top or bottom round, flank steak, tenderloin, or trimmed sirloin
> Lean lamb: center-cut lamb chops or lamb steaks
> Lean pork: center-cut pork chops, pork roast, ham, or Canadian bacon
> Lean veal: cutlets or center-cut veal chops

Poultry—Chicken, Turkey, and Game Hen

Poultry can be a healthy alternative to red meat because it is lower in fat. However, some poultry products, like wings, are high in fat. When shopping for a particular recipe that calls for ground beef, try substituting ground turkey (make sure the label reads "100% ground turkey breast"). Try to buy skinless poultry or remove the skin after cooking. When you're shopping, buy poultry you plan to grill, bake, broil, steam, or roast, not fry.

Seafood—Fish and Shellfish

Fish and seafood are usually healthy choices, as long as you avoid the types that are breaded and/or fried. It is important to prepare seafood so that it stays low fat and healthy, so shop for seafood recipes that involve baking, grilling, steaming, poaching, boiling, or broiling. Some tips for buying and keeping seafood fresh, healthy, and low fat:

- Always ask at the counter for the freshest choice.
- Be wary of fish with a strong fish odor or with eyes that look cloudy; it's probably not fresh.
- Purchase tuna packed in water.

Deli and Packaged Cold Cuts

Along the back wall is the packaged cold cuts section. The deli section will probably be separate and may be in the front or back of the store. In general, deli items and packaged cold cuts are high in fat and sodium, both of which we try to discourage in the DASH diet. There are now many reduced-fat or fat-free lunch meats, but these also may be high in sodium, so read the Nutrition Facts panel. You might be surprised to find that turkey or chicken franks are not always lower in fat than beef franks; again, it is important to read the label so you know what is going into your cart. The deli section will offer fresh cuts of ham, turkey, chicken, and lean roast beef, which are good alternatives to packaged meats.

Dairy Section
Milk and Yogurt

The back of the store usually also contains the dairy section, where you'll find the eggs, cheese, milk, buttermilk, and yogurt. Milk ranges in fat from 4% (whole milk) to 0% (skim milk). In between you can find ½%, 1%, or 2%. Buttermilk can be low fat or nonfat but contains more sodium. Some milk is fortified with calcium or protein. Remember that when cooking, you can replace cream with evaporated skim milk or one of the nonfat, nondairy substitutes.

Yogurt is an excellent low-fat, high-calcium food choice. It comes in whole-milk, low-fat, and nonfat forms, sweetened with sugar or artificially sweetened. It can be fruited or flavored or simply plain, allowing you to add what you like in the way of fruits, nuts, and seeds.

If you have problems digesting milk and dairy products, you might have lactose intolerance (see page 95). Look for milk with lactic acid (such as Lactase), or you might find lactase enzyme supplements convenient to use.

Cheese

Cheese may be kept in the dairy section or in a separate counter near the dairy section. In general, cheese is high in fat, saturated fat, sodium, and calories. Low-fat or part-skim milk cheeses have about 50 to 80 calories per ounce. Look for the low-fat varieties with less than 5 grams of fat per ounce. Good choices include part-skim or low-fat ricotta, low-fat cottage cheese, part-skim mozzarella, or string cheese.

Margarine and Butter

Margarine is a non-animal-based product made from vegetable oils. It is lower in saturated fat than butter and has no cholesterol. But it contains trans fatty acids, which can raise the cholesterol levels in your blood. We recommend sticking with native vegetable oils whenever possible. You might want to try a sprinkle or spray-on type of butter substitute for seasoning. If you must use margarine, choose a softer tub-style margarine, which is lower in trans fatty acids. If you do choose butter for its flavor, use it in moderation.

Bread Aisle

The bread aisle usually offers a wide variety of breads, rolls, English muffins, pita pockets, and specialty products. In general, most breads are low in fat. To increase your fiber intake, choose those labeled "whole wheat" or "100% whole wheat." Other tips to make your bread choices DASH healthy:

- Choose breads, muffins, or rolls with 2 grams of fat or less per serving.
- Purchase breads and muffins that are made with bran, oat bran, or pea fiber and provide 2 to 3 grams of fiber per serving.
- Avoid high-fat breads, such as biscuits, croissants, doughnuts, and sweet rolls.

The Inner Aisles

The inner aisles are the land of impulse buying. The rationale is that you will purchase items here because they look good or are on special. If impulse buying is an unhealthy habit for you, shop from a list and *never* go shopping when you are hungry. The inner aisles generally contain foods that have undergone more processing as well, which in some cases makes them less healthy choices than their counterparts found on the perimeter.

Canned Fruits and Vegetables

Canned fruits and vegetables are often higher in sugar and always higher in sodium than their fresh counterparts. Frozen fruits (without added sugar) and vegetables are better choices than canned, but if there's no other option, canned fruits and vegetables are better than not eating produce at all. In any case, it's not a bad idea to have some canned or dried foods on hand for such situations as an extended power outage or extreme weather. Some tips for choosing healthy fruit juices, canned fruits and vegetables, and dried fruits:

- Look for "no-salt-added" canned vegetables.
- Select 100 percent pure canned or frozen juices.
- Steer clear of fruit drinks or punches that are primarily sugar, water, and fruit flavor.
- Look for fruit canned or frozen without sugar and in its own juice.

Canned Soups

Grocery stores offer many types of canned soup, including fast entrees like minestrone, split pea, and vegetable. These can be a good alternative when fresh or frozen vegetables are not available, but look for "no-salt-added" or sodium-reduced soups. Avoid cream-based soups or use skim milk or water to reconstitute the soup instead of whole milk or cream.

Beans and Peas

Legumes such as chickpeas and beans are an inexpensive source of protein and other important nutrients. They can add great variety to meals and expand your meatless meal choices. Dried, canned, or even frozen beans or peas are all healthy choices, although the canned versions will be the highest in sodium. If you choose canned beans, rinse them thoroughly under water to remove as much as half the sodium.

Pasta and Rice

Pasta and rice are good sources of complex carbohydrates. Whole-grain and yolk-free pastas and brown rice are the healthiest choices because they are the highest in fiber. Plan on using only half of the seasoning packet in seasoned rice or pasta. To minimize your fat consumption and increase your intake of vegetables, buy tomato-based sauces. Shop for sauces made from herbs and olive oil instead of butter or cream. Remember, it is always a good idea to check the label for sodium and fat content.

Vegetable Oils and Cooking Fats

Since all oils and fats have the same number of calories (9 calories per gram) and there are 5 grams of fat in just 1 teaspoon, use them in moderation. Most vegetable oils are rich in unsaturated fat, but your best choices are the monounsaturated oils—olive, canola, peanut, and avocado. Olive oils that are labeled "extra virgin" are the first pressing of the olives and are richer in flavor and darker in color. "Light" and "mild" oils are lighter in color or milder in flavor but have just as many calories, so don't be fooled. Better still, choose a nonstick vegetable cooking spray when sautéing or greasing a pan.

Salad Dressings, Mayonnaise, and Mayonnaise-Type Dressings

Most grocery stores offer a wide variety of salad dressings, mayonnaise, and mayonnaise-type dressings, which are either regular, reduced calorie ("lite"), or fat free. The lower-fat, lower-calorie, or fat-free versions are your best option. They also make excellent marinades for meat, poultry, seafood, and vegetables. If you choose a regular thick dressing, you can cut back on the fat by thinning it with skim milk, plain yogurt, or water. Another tip for reducing fat in oil-based salad dressings: pour off the oil that rises to the top of the bottle—the flavor stays in; the fat goes down the drain.

Hot and Cold Cereals

Both hot and cold cereals can be an excellent source of fiber. Look for the whole-grain versions to make the most nutritious choices. Most cereals have 1 to 2 grams of fat per serving, and some have no fat at all. To keep your sugar, fat, and sodium intake low, check the Nutrition Facts panel for specific amounts per serving. Try to choose cereals with at least 3 grams of fiber, less than 3 grams of fat, and less than 5 grams of sugar per serving.

Crackers and Cookies

The cracker and cookie aisle can be very confusing. Many products that are labeled low fat and fat free are not terrific nutritional choices. Despite being low in fat, these foods are generally not high in nutrition. Often extra sugar is added to replace the flavor and texture from fat, so that lower in fat does not mean lower in calories. Cookies that have not been fat reduced can contain 6 to 8 grams of fat (or more) *per cookie*. A typical cracker contains 3 or 4 grams of fat per serving, but some are higher in fat than others, such as butter cookies, Ritz crackers, and Triscuit crackers. When you read the ingredients label, watch for items like butter, coconut or palm oil, unspecified shortening, and vegetable shortening.

Frozen Foods

Frozen dinners can save time. A whole dinner can be pulled from the freezer, or several side dishes can be used to round out a meal. When you buy frozen entrees or vegetables, avoid breaded and fried options. For frozen dinners, look for full meals with less than 800 milligrams of sodium, 10 to 15 grams of fat, and about 400 to 600 calories. If you choose a 300-calorie meal, you might not be getting enough energy from it.

Supplement it with other foods, like a glass of milk and a whole wheat roll.

It's a good idea to have some frozen vegetables on hand to help round out meals when fresh vegetables aren't available or when you don't want to clean and prepare them. Frozen fruits and fruit juices, when processed without added sugar, are also good freezer staples. If you select lower-fat frozen desserts, they may be higher in sugar—so the calories may be the same. Check the Nutrition Facts panel for more information. In general, ice milk, sherbet, and low-fat frozen yogurt have less fat than ice cream.

Dining Out on DASH

Eating out is the norm for increasing numbers of Americans. Estimates are that more than half of all meals are eaten away from home for reasons of preference, convenience, or long-distance travel. Because eating out is done so often, it is important that it be done in a healthy way.

Unfortunately, restaurants—especially fast-food outlets—don't often emphasize those foods that are the foundation of the DASH diet, notably fruits, vegetables, and low-fat dairy products. Although dining out can pose challenges if you are trying to adhere to DASH eating guidelines, there are certainly things you can do to make your meals away from home as DASH friendly as possible.

When eating out, people tend to forget their healthy eating guidelines, so above all, remember that eating away from home is not a vacation from taking care of yourself. Follow the promise you made to yourself about lowering your blood pressure and improving your overall health by searching out restaurants that serve healthier fare. The Internet can be a valuable source for finding vegetarian and health-food restaurants in your area or at your travel destination. At regular restaurants, don't be embarrassed to make special requests, such as having the chef prepare the food with less fat or including more vegetables and less meat. If you choose to eat at a fast-food outlet, make sensible choices about which establishment to eat at and what you eat (see page 134, "Fast-Food Facts").

Here are some tips for staying healthy while dining out or eating on the road:

Plan ahead. Choose restaurants that offer nutritious choices. Watch out for the restaurants that offer only low-nutrient, high-calorie selections, and be wary of all-you-can-eat buffets. Try to remember: *Eating is to give your body the nourishment it needs, not to see how much it can take.*

Before you go into a restaurant or look at a menu, decide what kind of food you want to eat. If you're eating the DASH diet, your goal should be to find something to eat and/or drink that's rich in fruits, vegetables, and low-fat dairy.

Don't go into a restaurant ravenous, or you will just be tempted to overeat. If you are so hungry that you are starving or feel light-headed or dizzy, you should eat something before you go out. Have some pretzels, a piece of fruit, or a half cup of juice or skim milk before you leave home. If you are very hungry before heading out to eat, it's easy to eat half your calorie allowance in bread and butter before your meal even arrives, not leaving any room for DASH-appropriate choices, such as vegetables and fruit.

Call ahead. When you order airline tickets, ask for an in-flight meal that is low fat, low sodium, or vegetarian. When the beverage cart comes around, ask for a carton of 1% milk to wash down your meal.

Stack the odds in your favor. When you have a flight or train ride ahead of you, carry along some simple, nonperishable snacks, such as low-fat crackers or fruit, so you'll have something healthy to eat when you're hungry. Having healthy snacks to nibble on can also break the monotony of a long journey.

Balance your choices. If you know you are going to have a dinner that does not contain as many fruits and vegetables as you need to meet your DASH diet requirements, eat plenty of those foods during the day. Also be vigilant about your sodium intake during the day if you know your evening meal will be high in sodium (fast-food outlets are major culprits when it comes to loading their offerings with sodium, as are many Chinese, Mexican, and "soul food" restaurants).

Make smart choices. Select 1% milk or fruit juice instead of alcohol or soda during the beverage service on flights or at restaurants. Even though a salad bar may sound like a healthy choice, it can be a minefield of fat, calories, and sodium. Most offer high-fat dressings, and some serve pepperoni, bacon bits, hard-boiled eggs, high-sodium soups, and even puddings or other desserts. Stick to the vegetables; avoid the fatty, salty items; and choose a low-fat, low-sodium dressing.

Be moderate. Watch your portion sizes. Remember, unless you are going to a trendy spot that serves "spa" portions, what you are served in most restaurants is rarely a reasonably sized portion. Don't overindulge just because you are eating out. If you order an appetizer, choose a nutritious one, such as raw vegetables, steamed mussels, or shrimp cocktail. Avoid overly "meaty" appetizer selections, fried appetizers, or ones with heavy sauces or cheese. Remember that size-wise, a couple of appetizers can be a meal in itself.

Go easy on alcohol. Be cautious about your alcohol consumption. Alcohol can affect your judgment of how much you eat and lead you to overindulgence. Some people find alcohol to be a sensitive subject at social occasions—for example, when wine is served with dinner or the host orders a round of after-dinner drinks—but it is always acceptable to decline a drink. You should know that alcohol is full of empty calories and easily turns into fat and unwanted pounds. A glass of wine a day is good for most people, according to the American Heart Association, but it is best for everyone who chooses to drink to do so in moderation. Moderation is defined as one or two drinks a day (see "Limit Your Alcohol Consumption," page 54).

Watch how often you eat out. Eating out too often can pose problems no matter how much you know about foods. Restaurant foods just aren't prepared as healthfully as home-cooked foods. Unless you find a truly special restaurant that serves particularly healthy fare, try to limit dining out to a couple of times a week. If you must dine out more often, look for places that offer simpler fare, such as bagel or sandwich shops, salad bars, or vegetarian restaurants where you can order low-fat items.

Choose low-fat foods. Make your menu selections wisely. Look for clues that a food is low in fat and then ask your waiter questions to find out if, what kind, and how much fat is used in preparing dishes (see the guidelines in chapter 6).

Keep an open mind. When traveling, don't overlook the low-fat selections at grocery stores, supermarkets, and local farmer's markets. Check out their fresh breads, fruit, yogurt, and salad bar. A piece of fruit or a single serving of nonfat or low-fat yogurt is a simple low-fat food-to-go choice and fits right in if you're trying to eat the DASH way. You can load the yogurt with fruit and nuts. Some grocery stores provide a cooler full of cold single-serving juice bottles near their self-serve salad bar. Many supermarkets also feature extensive delis and bakeries that prepare sandwiches and salads to go. Look for the deli section's to-order sandwiches and ask the counter person to make you something healthy.

Fast-Food Facts

Most people assume fast food is off-limits, but the fact is that many fast-food restaurants offer healthy options (remember, even some fast-food restaurants will accommodate special requests, such as leaving off the mayo or special sauce on a fish sandwich). Use the accompanying chart to assess your favorite fast-food restaurants. As a general rule, if you need around 2,200 calories a day, your total fat intake for the day should be less than 70 grams and your sodium intake should be about 1,600 milligrams.

Fat and Sodium Content of Some Fast-Food Restaurant Items

	Calories	Fat (grams)	Sodium (milligrams)
McDonald's			
Big Mac	510	26	930
Large fries	448	22	291
Egg McMuffin	290	13	730
Chicken McNuggets	300	18	530
McGrilled Chicken Classic	250	3	510
Chunky Chicken Salad	160	5	320
Serves 1 percent milk	104	2	128
Burger King			
Croissan'wich with Bacon, Egg & Cheese	350	24	790
Whopper with cheese	730	46	1,300
Broiled Chicken Sandwich	200	10	110
Serves 2 percent milk	120	5	122
Wendy's			
Single with Everything	440	23	860
Junior Cheeseburger Deluxe	390	20	820
Baked Potato, Plain	310	0	25
with Broccoli and Cheese	460	14	440
Breaded Chicken Sandwich	450	20	740
Deluxe Garden Salad (without dressing)	110	6	320
Frosty Dairy Dessert, 12 oz.	340	10	200
Serves 2 percent milk	120	5	122

Taco Bell

Beef Mexi-Melt	266	15	689
Mexican Pizza	575	37	1,031
Light Burrito Supreme	350	8	*
Light Taco Salad, without chips	464	9	*
Light Soft Taco	180	5	*

Domino's Pizza

Hand-Tossed with Ham, 2 slices of 12"	362	10	1,143
Thin crust, cheese only, ⅓ of 12"	364	16	1,012
Thin crust, veggie, ⅓ of 12"	386	17	1,076
Deep Dish X-tra cheese and pepperoni, 2 slices of 12"	671	33	1,508

Pizza Hut

Medium Pan crust cheese, 1 slice	261	11	501
Thin'N Crispy crust veggie lover's pizza, 1 slice	186	7	545
Pan crust pepperoni lover's, 1 slice	332	17	777
Personal pan supreme	637	34	1,760

TCBY

½ cup plain frozen yogurt:*			
No sugar added	80	0	35
Nonfat	110	0	45
Regular	130	3	50

*Does not include toppings and sauces.

Eating the DASH Way:
Any Tom, Dick, or Harriet Can Do It

By using the food groups and serving suggestions, you can figure out how to eat the DASH way without too much trouble
at all. To emphasize the point that this is a relatively easy diet
to adopt, we'll present how three different people might eat
the DASH way and, if they were just starting the DASH diet,
how they would keep track. You can photocopy the form on
pages 142–143 to keep track yourself.

Tom

"Tom," thirty-one years old, is a conductor on a San Francisco
trolley. He is 5 feet 11 inches tall and weighs 175 pounds. He
spends a good portion of his day on his feet and also walks
recreationally on his days off.

Tom wakes at six in the morning and watches the news on
TV as he sits down to a breakfast consisting of a glass of 100
percent apple juice, a bowl of bran cereal served with skim
milk, and a handful of raisins. He also has a slice of his favorite
whole-wheat toast, which he eats with margarine. Before he
heads out the door, he packs himself a bag lunch—a chicken
sandwich on whole-wheat bread with low-fat American
cheese, lettuce, tomato, and "light" mayonnaise. He also slips
an apple, a bag of unsalted pretzels, and a bottle of water into
his lunchbox. On his way to the trolley depot, he picks himself
up a large coffee made with skim milk, to which he adds two
packets of a nonsugar sweetener. A couple of hours after eating
his bag lunch, Tom ducks into a convenience store during his
break and for a midday snack buys a banana and a carton of
100 percent orange juice. When it's time to go home for dinner, Tom makes a point of stopping at the supermarket to buy
a simple but tasty salad to go with the spaghetti dinner he's

Food	Amount	Servings Provided	
		Vegetables	Fruits
Breakfast			
apple juice	1 cup		1 1/2
bran cereal, ready-to-eat	2/3 cup		
raisins	2 Tbsp.		1/2
skim milk	1 cup		
whole-wheat bread	2 slices		
soft margarine	1 tsp.		
Lunch			
chicken sandwich:			
chicken breast (no skin)	3 oz.		
American cheese reduced fat	2 slices (1 1/2 oz.)		
loose-leaf lettuce	2 large leaves	1/2	
tomato	2 slices (1/4" thick)	1/2	
light mayonnaise	1 Tbsp.		
whole-wheat bread	2 slices		
apple	1 medium		1
pretzel, unsalted	1 cup		
Dinner			
vegetarian spaghetti sauce*	3/4 cup	1 1/2	
spaghetti	1 1/2 cups		
Parmesan cheese, grated	3 Tbsp.		
green beans	1 cup	2	
spinach salad: spinach raw	1 1/2 cups	1 1/2	
mushrooms, raw	1/4 cup	1/4	
croutons	2 Tbsp.		
Italian dressing, low-fat	2 Tbsp.		
dinner roll	2 medium		
soft margarine	1 tsp.		
frozen yogurt, low-fat	1/2 cup		
Snacks			
orange juice	1 cup		1 1/2
banana	1 large		1 1/2
Day's Totals		**6 1/4**	**6**

*See page 204.

Servings Provided

Dairy foods	Grains	Meat, poultry, and fish	Nuts, seeds, and legumes	Added fats and oils	Sweets
	1				
1					
	2				
				1	
		1			
1					
				1	
	2				
	1				
	3				
1					
	1/4				
				1	
	2				
				1	
1					
4	**11 1/4**	**1**	**0**	**4**	**0**

planning to make (the salad he makes up contains spinach, raw mushrooms, croutons, and low-fat Italian dressing). That night he has his spaghetti dinner made with linguine and a store-bought vegetarian spaghetti sauce. Tom usually drinks water with his meals, but this evening he has a glass of wine as a "reward" for the fact that he has been diligent about eating lots of fruits, vegetables, and low-fat dairy products and has cut back on the number of burgers he eats every week.

Pages 138–139 shows how Tom would have filled out the self-tracking form shown on pages 142–143.

Dick

"Dick" is fifty-two years old and works in a bank in a small midwestern town. He is 5 feet 7 inches tall and weighs 160 pounds.

For breakfast Dick has a cup of prune juice, half a cup of oatmeal topped with a sliced whole banana, a slice of whole-wheat toast with a teaspoon of soft margarine, and a cup of skim milk.

For lunch he hits a deli near the bank, where he knows Marge, the woman who makes the sandwiches. In contrast to the bologna, white bread, and mayo sandwich he often used to eat, Dick has started asking Marge to make him a low-sodium lean-meat ham or turkey sandwich on whole-wheat bread, topped with two slices of reduced-fat cheese, two leaves of lettuce, two slices of tomato, and mustard (he tells Marge to "go easy on the meat and put on plenty of lettuce and tomato instead"). Surprised as Marge is about Dick's healthier new choices, she has started eating better herself and has posted Dick's choice on the chalkboard behind the counter as the "Heart-Healthy Sandwich of the Day." On the way to the checkout counter, Dick picks up an apple and a diet soda and then heads to a park bench on the town common, where he eats his lunch before going back to the office.

Feeling a little hungry by midafternoon, Dick helps himself to a few dried apricots and unsalted almonds he keeps in a plastic bag in his top drawer.

Dick gets home at 5:30 after stopping at the supermarket to pick up a couple of ingredients for the dinner that his wife, Lisa, is making. While Lisa prepares dinner, Dick peels and eats an orange and helps his youngest son with his homework. Lisa makes chicken and Spanish rice, which she serves with green peas and a piece of corn bread. Everyone at the table drinks a glass of skim milk and enjoys melon balls for dessert.

Harriet

"Harriet" is a thirty-year-old nurse practitioner who lives by herself in Boston and is engaged to be married. She is 5 feet 9 inches, weighs 160 pounds, and stays in great shape by biking to and from work when weather permits and going to the gym at least five times a week.

At 5:30 in the morning Harriet bikes to the hospital where she works. Before heading to her office, she buys breakfast in the hospital cafeteria and eats it while she reviews her notes from the day before and plans the day's schedule. Her choices this morning: a carton of orange juice, a cup of fat-free yogurt, two low-fat granola bars, a banana, and a cup of skim milk. Unable to finish this hearty meal, she saves the banana for a mid-morning snack.

After a hectic morning's work, it's time for lunch. Harriet—eager to get away from the hospital for just a few moments—meets up with a friend and pops over to a local lunch spot that has an excellent salad bar. There she buys a large salad heavy on romaine lettuce, mushrooms, chickpeas, and a bonanza of other veggies, which she dresses with balsamic vinaigrette. She also buys a whole-wheat roll and washes the whole lot down with a carton of skim milk. Dessert is an apple. That night Harriet goes out for dinner with one of her bridesmaids-

Food	Amount	Servings Provided	
		Vegetables	Fruits
Breakfast			
Lunch			
Dinner			
Snacks			
Day's Totals			
Compare yours with the Dash plan		4–5	4–5

to-be. They choose an Italian restaurant near where Harriet lives. Harriet selects a penne pasta dish served with a vegetarian fresh plum tomato sauce. The restaurant is known for its large portions, so ahead of time Harriet promises herself she'll eat only half of what she is served and take the rest home with her to heat up for lunch tomorrow at the hospital. She has two slices of the bread the waiter serves before the meal arrives but

Servings Provided

Dairy foods	Grains	Meat, poultry, and fish	Nuts, seeds, and legumes	Added fats and oils	Sweets
2–3	7–8	2	4–5	2–3	5 a week

skips the butter and instead lightly dabs her bread in a flavored olive oil provided at the table. Harriet and her friend
share a salad but skip dessert at the restaurant because all the
choices seem to be high in fat. After dinner the two young
women go to a local ice cream outlet, where Harriet buys a
small fat-free frozen yogurt topped with nuts.

Track Your Food Habits

Self-monitoring is one of the most effective ways to ensure the success of a healthful change in behavior. Use the form on pages 142–143 to track your food habits before you start on the DASH eating plan and to see how you're doing after a few weeks. To record more than one day, just copy the form. Total each day's food groups and compare what you ate with the DASH plan. To see how the form looks completed, see pages 138–139.

8

———————∨———————

Make DASH Part of
Your Life . . . for Life!

Wouldn't it be wonderful if we could make positive lifestyle changes quickly and easily and keep up our new, healthier behaviors for the rest of our lives? The truth is, beginning and maintaining improvements in how we eat isn't easy for most of us.

Even DASH—an easy-to-understand, nondeprivation eating system made up of familiar foods—can be difficult to adhere to if you don't have a plan.

You may have taken the 14-Day DASH challenge and discovered that your blood pressure went down significantly and you felt great. After your doctor gave you the news about your blood pressure, you were probably excited that you had found a direct and immediate way to lower your blood pressure. But what do you do when your initial enthusiasm wanes and old tastes and habits resurface? What happens if your spouse or kids insist on having doughnuts in your newly cleared fridge? Or if the local fast-food joint is oh-so-convenient on the way home from work? Or you feel like going out and buying a whole pint of ice cream to eat on the couch because you are stressed?

The point is that nutrition knowledge isn't enough. You have to confront your eating behaviors and gain skills to deal with the challenges of eating more healthfully.

Our team of expert nutritionists has helped thousands of people improve their eating behaviors. Over the years they have developed a program of key steps that you can use to start and stick with the DASH diet.

Step 1: Recognize Your Food Issues

Understand your relationship with food and decide what you need to change to follow the DASH diet.

Consider whether any of the following are issues for you, or add your own food issue:

    not eating enough fruits, vegetables, or low-fat dairy
        products
    eating too many fats and sugars
    eating while watching TV
    late-night eating
    eating out at fast-food outlets too often
    eating too much
    eating too fast
    eating too many processed foods

Step 2: Believe You Will Succeed

You can make big changes in the long term by working on one or two behavioral steps at a time.

If you have tried to improve your diet many times before and not succeeded—as have millions of Americans before you—you may feel you have failed or that you are a failure. The step-by-step approach in this chapter is one that encourages you to make smaller changes so you can succeed one step at a time.

Remember that you are unique—a person with your own strengths and weaknesses. Don't compare yourself with others. What works for someone else may not be right for you. The challenge is to find what does work for you. If you want to, you *can* learn and change. Setting realistic and achievable goals will help you succeed (see step 5, below).

Step 3: Time It Right

Are you ready to make the commitment?

Eating the DASH way—indeed, making any lifestyle change—is something that you have to do *for yourself*, although you do not always have to do it by yourself. No one can do it for you. Sometimes loving family members or concerned health professionals push people to make changes for which they aren't ready. Unless you are ready to make a commitment to work on your own nutrition and health, your chances for success are limited.

Timing is important, because real change takes perseverance and commitment and often you have to make a number of attempts before things start to work. That is okay. The only sure way *not* to succeed is never to try!

Step 4: One Step Leads You to the Next

Making changes is a process, and you will continue to learn as you go.

When you start the DASH diet, you won't know everything about nutrition—or yourself. Thus begins a great learning opportunity! Every eating event is a chance to gain insight into how and why you eat. Reflect on your experiences, your eating patterns, and your habits and then move on from there.

This process takes you from self-awareness to learning and using skills to make actual changes in your life. Skills are a necessary step for making changes. Consider which skills you need to develop to help you eat the DASH way:

- Learn what the serving sizes are for each of the food groups.
- Master healthier cooking techniques
- Choose healthier snacking options.
- Modify recipes so they are healthier.
- Read food labels.
- Practice more sensible dining-out routines.
- Avoid and cope with eating "triggers."

Step 5: Develop a SMART Action Plan

Break the task into specific, small, behavioral steps.

Changing your diet involves several different behaviors. Goal setting is an ongoing process. Use the SMART approach, below, to help you succeed and avoid getting frustrated. By SMART we mean recognizing that small, specific steps are the best way to move toward larger goals.

The SMART Approach

Specific: Make your goal very specific; for example, say "I will eat more than five servings each of fruits and vegetables every day" instead of "I will try to eat more fruits and vegetables."

Measurable: You can track your progress if your goal is measurable; for example, say "I will add up the total number of servings of fruits and vegetables each night to make sure I am eating as much as the DASH diet recommends."

Action Oriented: To change, you must act, *do something*; for example, say "I will eat more fruits and vegetables and keep a written record of the number of servings *every time* I eat during the next week."

Realistic: Goals that are not realistic are seldom reached. Work on small changes that you can really do. Fortunately, the DASH diet is a realistic diet that you *can* really do.

Timed: Give yourself a definite timetable for your specific action; for example, after successfully sticking with your goal of five servings each of fruits and vegetables for two weeks, you can set a new goal of limiting your intake of meat to two servings per day.

Step 6: "Just Do It"

To get anywhere, you have to start somewhere!

The time and effort spent planning and thinking about the changes you need to make do no good unless you act. *Doing* your new behaviors may feel like a lot of effort in the beginning but with practice will become easier. This is the crucial step where at times you have to give yourself that extra push! This is where you use your commitment to yourself to go ahead and *do* even though you may not feel like it; for example, "When I feel like going for fast food instead of taking the time to eat from the supermarket salad bar, I *will make* time knowing that I'll feel good about my choice once I've done it."

Step 7: Assess Your Progress

Reassess where you are now and where you've come from.

One of the most effective ways to ensure your efforts at changing your behavior are successful is to monitor yourself. Self-monitoring means keeping track of what you're doing to change your behavior. When it comes to eating the DASH diet, this means counting the number of servings you're eating from each of the food groups to see how close you are to your goals. DASH is easier to keep track of than many diets, but you may need to write things down until you get good at it. Use the tracing form on pages 142–143 and be diligent about filling it out every day—better still, after every meal—until eating the DASH diet becomes second nature.

There are other ways to keep track of your progress. Find what works comfortably for you. You can choose to use a number of different monitoring tools and objective measures. Consider any of the following suggestions:

- Periodically check portion sizes using measuring cups and spoons.
- Keep a journal to monitor general progress and difficulties.
- Note positive changes, such as blood pressure readings.
- Follow other medical data, such as blood sugar, cholesterol, heart rate.
- Check your progress on the calendar.
- Put money in a glass jar for every step accomplished.

Step 8: Ask for Help If Things Aren't Going Well

You don't have to go it alone.

These are some of the ways to get support:

- Ask for help from family, friends, co-workers, minister, or health professional.
- Find a "DASH buddy" to work along with you.
- Work on relaxation techniques.
- Join or form a support group.
- Look at the specific steps in your action plan and establish other specific steps.
- Take a break and do something that is fun.
- Don't expect things to always run smoothly.
- Read material that is helpful.

And the Final Step: Celebrate Every Success,
No Matter How Small!

Perhaps you are often too ambitious, impatient, or hard on yourself. Give yourself credit for the steps you have mastered on the way. *Every* small step is a real move in the right direction, and you deserve to feel good about your hard work. Of course, the challenge is to celebrate in a way that fits with your greater goals. If food has been your way of rewarding yourself, you may want to explore other ways to feel good. It is *very* important to feel good because when you do, you'll be able to accomplish so much more for yourself.

PART FOUR

———————⋀———————

DASH Menu Plans
and Recipes

9

——————／\——————

Fourteen Days on the DASH Diet

In this chapter you'll find two weeks of DASH diet menu plans. To create them, a team of DASH nutritionists used sophisticated computer technology to ensure that the nutrient content of the meals would add up to the amounts we proved would lower blood pressure.

We provide these menu plans so that you can make lifestyle changes completely and without delay and get started immediately on the DASH diet. These menu plans also let you begin right away on the "14-day DASH diet challenge" (see page 9).

There are other advantages to thinking in advance about what foods to assemble for a meal, a day, or a week:

It saves time and effort. Needed items will be on hand, which means fewer trips to the grocery store. Planning helps you make good use of leftovers, which can decrease preparation time and food costs.

It saves money. When you go to the store, you will know what you need. Then you can compare prices and buy only what you can use without waste. Preplanned quick meals can replace more costly convenience items and restaurant meals at least some of the time.

It increases variety. You can include the foods you need for nutrients and dietary fiber, such as whole grains, vegetables, fruits, and low-fat dairy products. You can also include new food items, try new styles of preparation occasionally, and vary the colors, textures, flavors, and shapes of foods to make meals attractive and interesting.

It helps you stick to the DASH diet. You can balance your food choices to increase your consumption of fruits, vegetables, and low-fat dairy foods and restrict how much fat, sugar, and sodium you are eating.

The menus are flexible and can be used in any order. You can also exchange a meal from one day's menu with a meal from the same part of the menu from another day (a lunch for a lunch and so forth). You can also substitute a meal from the recipes provided in chapter 10. Combining a breakfast, lunch, dinner, and snack from anywhere in the two weeks of menu plans will provide you with the total recommended daily number of servings from the food groups.

Meeting Your Calorie-Intake Requirement

The menu plans in this chapter are for a person whose daily calorie intake is between 1,800 and 2,200 calories. That's most of us. You may have a different calorie-intake requirement, but it is easy to adapt the menu plans to fit your needs.

If your calorie-intake requirement is outside the 1,800–2,200 range, you will need to eat different numbers of servings from the ones given in the menu plans in this chapter.* You can find out how many servings you should eat for your calorie-intake requirement by referring to the table on page 80. For example, if your calorie-intake requirement is 2,800 calories a day (within the 2,600–3,000 calorie-intake range), then *compared to someone eating a 2,000-calorie diet,* you need to

---

*If you don't know what your calorie-intake requirements are, refer to pages 78–79.

eat an additional two servings each of fruits and vegetables, one more serving of low-fat dairy products, two more servings of grains, and one more serving of meat every day. You can also allow yourself one and a half additional daily servings of sweets and two more servings of added fats and oils. To increase the number of servings from a particular food group, you can either add a different item from within that food group to your meal or simply increase the serving size of the item you are already planning to eat.

Our tables don't go any higher than 3,000 calories, but some people may need to eat more than this amount. If you are one of them, follow this simple guideline: for every 500 calories you need to eat in excess of 3,000 calories, add another serving each of vegetables, fruits, and grains and half a serving each of low-fat dairy and meat.

The key to adapting the 2,000-calorie menu plans given here to your own calorie-intake requirement is to proportionally increase or decrease all food groups. As far as possible, when *increasing* calorie intake to meet your requirements, focus on those food groups that are *less* dense in energy (vegetables, fruits, and grains), and when *decreasing* calorie intake, focus on those food groups that are *more* dense in energy (meats, added fats and oils, and sweets).

How the Menu Plans Break Down

DASH nutritionists used state-of-the-art computer technology to calculate the exact nutrient content of the menu plans in this chapter. However, the basic framework of each day's meals can be broken down quite simply:

Meals	Recommended Servings	Example Pattern
Breakfast	Fruits (2 servings)	Any fresh fruits/juices
	Dairy (1 serving)	Skim milk
	Grains (2 servings)	Ready-to-eat cereals
Lunch	Vegetables (2 servings)	Any vegetables
	Fruits (1 serving)	Any fruits/juices
	Dairy (1 serving)	Sandwich with lean
	Grains (2 servings)	meat and reduced-
	Meat (½ serving)	fat cheese
Dinner	Vegetables (3 servings)	Any vegetables
	Fruits (1 serving)	Fruit juice
	Dairy (1 serving)	Skim milk
	Grains (2 servings)	Cooked grains
		(pasta, rice, etc.)
	Meat (1 serving)	Fish or meat
Snack	Grains (1 serving)	Unsalted light
		popcorn
	Nuts/seeds (½ serving)	Any unsalted nuts

This is one example of achieving the suggested food groups. You can always structure your daily diet differently.

Snacking on the DASH Diet

The DASH diet is a hearty eating plan. However, if you find you are still hungry or you like to eat between meals, consider healthy snacking. When snacking as an addition to the DASH diet, choose from among the grain and nut groups. If you find the DASH diet substantial enough and want to cut a fruit, vegetable, or dairy product from one of your meals, eat whatever you cut from your meal as a snack.

These are some examples of snacks from the grain and nut food groups. Choose a total of one per day.

100 *calories each*

3 graham crackers
6 low-fat vanilla wafers
10 unsalted pretzels
3 cups plain popcorn (with a touch of butter flavoring)
1 ounce baked potato chips

200 *calories each*

¼ cup unsalted roasted nuts, such as cashews, peanuts, mixed nuts, walnuts, or almonds

Week 1: 2,000-Calorie Menus

	Monday	Tuesday	Wednesday	Thursday
B R E A K F A S T	1 cup apple juice 3 tablespoons raisins ⅔ cup shredded wheat 1 cup skim milk 1 slice whole-wheat toast 1 teaspoon unsalted margarine 1 teaspoon jelly	½ cup prunes ½ cup strawberries 1 cup cooked oatmeal 1 slice whole-wheat toast 1 teaspoon unsalted margarine 1 cup skim milk	1 cup orange juice ½ cup cantaloupe cubes ½ whole-wheat bagel 2 teaspoons jelly 1 tablespoon fat-free cream cheese 1 cup skim milk	1 cup orange juice ¼ cup banana slices ¼ cup strawberries 1 English muffin, toasted 1 tablespoon almond butter 8 ounces nonfat yogurt
L U N C H	1 serving Broccoli and Walnut Salad* with: 4 slices tomato 6 pieces romaine lettuce 1 whole-wheat pita pocket ¾ cup plain nonfat yogurt ¾ cup pineapple tidbits	1 Hawaiian Chicken Sandwich* 1 serving Tomato and Red Onion Salad* 1 serving Smoothie*	Roast Beef Sandwich: 2 ounces roast beef, trimmed 2 slices mixed-grain bread 1 teaspoon low-sodium barbecue sauce ½ cup chopped romaine ½ cup chopped tomatoes ¼ cup chopped green peppers 1 tablespoon low-sodium diet Italian salad dressing 1 baked potato 1 medium apple 1 cup skim milk	Chicken Sandwich: 2 ounces chicken breast 2 slices whole-wheat bread 1½ ounces low sodium cheddar cheese 2 slices tomato ¼ cup shredded iceberg lettuce 10 baby carrots ¾ cup applesauce 1 medium banana

*Recipes for asterisked items can be found in chapter 10.

Friday	Saturday	Sunday
1 cup orange juice 1 medium peach 2 oatmeal-raisin granola bars 1 slice whole-wheat toast 1 teaspoon unsalted margarine 1 cup skim milk	1 cup orange juice ½ cup cantaloupe cubes 1 cinnamon-raisin bagel 1 tablespoon fat-free cream cheese 1 tablespoon orange marmalade 1 cup skim milk	1 cup orange juice ½ medium grapefruit 2 servings Blueberry Pancakes* 1 tablespoon maple syrup 1 cup skim milk
Tuna Fish Sandwich: 2 ounces tuna, water packed, unsalted 2 slices whole-wheat bread 2 teaspoons low-sodium light mayonnaise 2 slices tomato 2 ounces low-sodium, low-fat cheese 3 pieces romaine lettuce ½ cup steamed broccoli 1 medium peach	Chicken Sandwich: 2 ounces roasted chicken breast 2 slices whole-wheat bread 2 tablespoons low-sodium light mayonnaise 3 pieces romaine lettuce 2 slices tomato 10 baby carrots 1 orange 1 cup skim milk 1 Jell-O gelatin snack	Chicken Salad: ¼ cup chopped cooked chicken breast 2 teaspoons low-sodium light mayonnaise ¼ cup shredded lettuce 2 slices tomato ⅛ cup sliced red onion ¼ cup alfalfa sprouts ½ whole-wheat pita pocket 1 serving Sweet-Potato Chips* 1 medium banana 1 cup skim milk

Week 1: 2,000-Calorie Menus

	Monday	Tuesday	Wednesday	Thursday
D I N N E R	1 serving Dave's Cajun Catfish* ½ serving New Orleans Red Beans and Rice* ½ cup steamed okra 2 servings Lighter Sweet Country Corn Bread* 1 serving Tossed Salad I or Tossed Salad II* 1 teaspoon olive oil 1 tablespoon balsamic vinegar ½ medium fresh papaya 1 cup skim milk	1 serving Blackened Beef with Greens and Red Potatoes* 2 slices whole-wheat bread 1 cup plain nonfat yogurt ½ cup fruit cocktail	1 serving grilled Tuna* 1 serving Wild Rice Pilaf* 1 serving Sautéed Collard Greens* 10 baby carrots 1 tablespoon fat-free ranch salad dressing 1 serving Baked Apple* 2 whole-wheat rolls 2 teaspoons unsalted margarine 1 cup skim milk	1½ cups Gingered Butternut Soup* 1½ cups Tossed Salad I or Tossed Salad II* 2 cherry tomatoes 2 tablespoons salt-free French salad dressing 2 whole-wheat rolls 2 tablespoons shredded low-sodium cheddar cheese 2 teaspoons unsalted margarine 1 cup orange juice

*Recipes for asterisked items can be found in chapter 10.

Friday	Saturday	Sunday
1 serving Baked Catfish*	1 serving Fettuccine with Chicken and Vegetables*	1 serving Grilled Tuna*
1 serving Red Potato and Spinach Salad*	1 serving Soybean Salad*	1 serving Bulgar Wheat with Tomatoes*
½ cup steamed broccoli	1 cup steamed green beans	1 serving Sautéed Collard Greens*
2 whole-wheat rolls	2 slices Italian bread	1 serving Quick Pumpkin Bread*
2 teaspoons unsalted margarine	1 teaspoon unsalted margarine	½ cup plain low-fat yogurt
1 cup vanilla low-fat yogurt	¼ cup cantaloupe cubes	1 cup applesauce
1 medium peach	¼ cup papaya cubes	
	¼ cup banana slices	
	½ cup low-fat frozen yogurt	

Week 2: 2,000-Calorie Menus

	Monday	Tuesday	Wednesday	Thursday
B R E A K F A S T	1 cup orange juice 1 egg, poached or boiled 1 Lemon Muffin* 1 medium banana 1 cup skim milk	1 cup apple juice ⅔ cup shredded wheat 3 tablespoons raisins 1 slice whole-wheat toast 1 teaspoon unsalted margarine 1 teaspoon jelly 1 cup skim milk	1 cup orange juice ½ cup raspberries ¾ cup Frosted Mini Wheats 1 cup skim milk 1 slice whole-wheat toast 1 teaspoon unsalted margarine	½ cup prunes ½ cup strawberries 1 cup cooked oatmeal 1 slice whole-wheat toast 1 teaspoon unsalted margarine 1 cup skim milk
L U N C H	1 serving Couscous with Broccoli* 1 serving Quick Pumpkin Bread* 1 cup skim milk 1 medium banana	1 cup apple juice 1 serving Tomato-Orange Soup* 1 cup steamed green beans 2 whole-wheat rolls 1 teaspoon unsalted margarine 2 medium plums ½ cup skim milk	1 cup orange juice 1 serving Wild Rice Pilaf* 2 tablespoons low-sodium cheddar cheese 1 cup steamed mixed vegetables ½ cup frozen yogurt	1 cup orange juice 1 Swiss Cheese Sandwich* ½ cup watermelon balls

*Recipes for asterisked items can be found in chapter 10.

Friday	Saturday	Sunday
1 cup orange juice 1 serving Apple Cobbler* 1 slice whole-wheat toast 1 teaspoon unsalted margarine 1 cup skim milk	1 cup orange juice 2 Blueberry pancakes* 1 tablespoon maple syrup 1 cup skim milk ½ medium grapefruit	1 cup orange juice ¾ cup Frosted Mini Wheats 1 cup skim milk ½ cup raspberries 1 slice whole-wheat bread 1 teaspoon unsalted margarine
1 serving Tossed Salad Greens* 1 serving Tortellini and Bean Soup* 1 whole-wheat roll 1 serving Chocolate-Dipped Fruit* 1 cup skim milk	1 serving Turkey Burger* 1 serving Coleslaw with Dates* 1 medium apple 1 cup skim milk	1 cup apple juice 1 serving Tomato-Orange Soup* 2 whole-wheat rolls 1 teaspoon unsalted margarine 1 cup steamed green beans 2 plums ½ cup skim milk

Week 2: 2,000-Calorie Menus

	Monday	Tuesday	Wednesday	Thursday
D I N N E R	1 serving Snapper with Greens* ½ serving Fresh Fruit Salad* 1 baked potato 2 tablespoons salsa 2 tablespoons plain low-fat yogurt 2 whole-wheat rolls ½ cup citrus fruit sorbet	1 serving Sweet-and-Sour Pork with Vegetables* 1 cup cooked brown rice 1 serving Cherry Tomato and Scallion Salad* 2 teaspoons fresh lemon juice 1 serving Vanilla Pudding with Banana* ½ cup skim milk	1 serving Chicken Fruity Stir-fry* ½ cup cooked brown rice ½ cup steamed green peas 1 serving Stuffed Acorn Squash* ¾ cup plain nonfat yogurt ½ banana	1 cup orange juice 1 serving Northeast Gumbo* 1 cup cooked brown rice 1 serving Tossed Salad I or Tossed Salad II* 1 teaspoon olive oil 1 tablespoon balsamic vinegar 3 tablespoons shredded cheddar cheese 1 serving Apple Crisp*

*Recipes for asterisked items can be found in chapter 10.

Friday	Saturday	Sunday
1 serving Vermont Roast* 1 serving Baked Brown Bread* 1 serving Tossed Salad I or Tossed Salad II* 1 teaspoon olive oil 1 tablespoon balsamic vinegar 1 cup vanilla low-fat frozen yogurt ½ cup strawberries	½ cup orange juice 1 serving Baked Macaroni and Cheese* 1 serving Tossed Salad I or Tossed Salad II* 1 tablespoon low-sodium French dressing 1 serving Green Beans with Almonds* 2 whole-wheat rolls 1 teaspoon unsalted margarine 1 serving Orange-Banana Fruit Salad*	4 ounces salmon fillet 1 cup cooked brown rice 1 serving Three Bean Salad* 1 serving Broccoli Rabe* 1 serving Lighter Sweet Country Corn Bread* 1 serving Smoothie*

10

⟋\⟍

DASH Recipes

The following 67 recipes were created by a team of DASH nutritionists, and many of them are included in the two weeks of menu plans provided in chapter 9. These recipes show you how to prepare tasty, hearty meals that meet the DASH recommendations. Serve these recipes with the other foods listed in the menu plans or in dishes you have created yourself using the guidelines in this book.

Each recipe lists the following:

- ingredients and preparation instructions
- the number of servings it will make
- the number of servings of each food group in an individual portion
- the calories, total fat, fat, and sodium in a serving

Main Dishes

Baked Catfish

Baked Macaroni and Cheese

BBQ Pork Chops

Blackened Beef with Greens and Red Potatoes

Chicken and Broccoli Bake

Chicken Fruity Stir-fry

Chicken with Rice

Dave's Cajun Catfish

Fettuccine with Chicken and Vegetables

Grilled Tuna

Hawaiian Chicken Sandwich

*Mango and Black Bean Salad
with Grilled Shrimp*

New Orleans Red Beans and Rice

Northeast Gumbo

Snapper with Greens

Main Dishes (cont.)

Spicy Cod

Sweet-and-Sour Pork with Vegetables

Swiss Cheese Sandwich

Turkey Burger

Vegetarian Lasagna

Vegetarian Spaghetti Sauce

Vermont Roast with Brown Mustard

DASH-Sodium Results Are In . . . so Salt Is Out

An important note: The recipes given here are reduced in salt, to match the combination of DASH diet plus salt reduction that was particularly effective in the DASH-Sodium study (see chapter 4). The reason for this is simple: we wanted to make it easy for you to use the diet that has worked best at lowering blood pressure. The DASH diet will lower blood pressure without reducing salt, but not as well.

Baked Catfish

⅓ cup all-purpose flour
⅓ cup dried bread crumbs
1½ teaspoons paprika
Pinch of freshly ground black
    pepper

2 tablespoons grated
    Parmesan cheese
2 pounds catfish fillets
¾ cup plain nonfat yogurt

Preheat the oven to 450°F. Mix the flour, bread crumbs, paprika, pepper, and Parmesan. Cut the fish into 5-ounce pieces. Coat with the yogurt and dredge in the flour/crumb mixture. Place on sheet pans lightly sprayed with nonstick cooking spray. Bake for 10 minutes.

Servings	Calories per serving	Fat (g)	Sodium (mg)
6 (5 ounces each)	216	5	173

	Vegetables	Fruits/Juices	Dairy Foods	Grains
Food Group Serving(s):				

	Meat, Poultry, and Fish	Nuts, Seeds, and Legumes	Added Fats/Oils	Sweets
Food Group Serving(s):	1			

Baked Macaroni and Cheese

———————⋀———————

2 cups dried macaroni

2 tablespoons stick margarine

4 teaspoons minced onion

1 tablespoon all-purpose flour

¼ teaspoon dry mustard

⅛ teaspoon ground white
    pepper

2 cups skim milk

8 ounces grated 50% reduced-
    fat cheddar cheese

2 ripe tomatoes, thinly sliced

1 teaspoon dried parsley
    flakes

Cook the macaroni according to label directions. While the
macaroni is cooking, preheat the oven to 400°F. Melt the
margarine in a saucepan over medium-high heat. Add the
onion, flour, dry mustard, and white pepper to the pan.
Slowly stir in the milk. Cook, stirring frequently, until smooth
and hot, about 8 minutes.

Add the cheese to the pan and stir just until it is melted,
about 10 seconds. When the macaroni is tender, drain in a
colander and transfer to a 2-quart casserole. Pour the cheese
sauce over the macaroni and toss lightly to mix. Arrange
tomato slices on top of the macaroni and sauce. Sprinkle the
parsley over the tomatoes. Bake, uncovered, in the preheated
oven for 20 minutes.

Servings	Calories per serving	Fat (g)	Sodium (mg)
6 (1 cup each)	309	11	321

	Vegetables	Fruits/Juices	Dairy Foods	Grains
Food Group Serving(s):	1		1	1

	Meat, Poultry, and Fish	Nuts, Seeds, and Legumes	Added Fats/Oils	Sweets
Food Group Serving(s):				

BBQ Pork Chops

1 (10-ounce) can low-sodium
tomato soup

2 tablespoons Worcestershire
sauce

3 tablespoons red wine
vinegar

4 tablespoons dehydrated
minced onion

1 teaspoon paprika

1 teaspoon chili powder

¾ cup water

¼ teaspoon ground cinnamon

⅛ teaspoon ground cloves

⅛ teaspoon freshly ground
black pepper

1½ pounds boneless top loin
pork chops, trimmed of all
fat

Combine all the ingredients except the pork chops in a large bowl. Transfer to a skillet with high sides, add the pork chops, and simmer over medium heat for 30 to 40 minutes. (The pork chops may also be cut into cubes before cooking.) Serve each pork chop over ⅔ cup of cooked rice.

Servings	Calories per serving	Fat (g)	Sodium (mg)
6 (4 ounces each) without rice	254	13	120

	Vegetables	Fruits/Juices	Dairy Foods	Grains
Food Group Serving(s):				

	Meat, Poultry, and Fish	Nuts, Seeds, and Legumes	Added Fats/Oils	Sweets
Food Group Serving(s):	1			

Blackened Beef with Greens and Red Potatoes

————————⌄————————

1 pound lean top round of
  beef

2 tablespoons paprika

1 tablespoon dried oregano

1 teaspoon chili powder

½ teaspoon garlic powder

½ teaspoon freshly ground
  black pepper

¼ teaspoon cayenne pepper

¼ teaspoon dry mustard

6 medium red potatoes cut
  into quarters about 1 inch
  thick (about 6 cups)

3 cups finely chopped onions

2 cups beef broth

2 cups water

2 cloves garlic, minced

3 large carrots, cut into
  rounds about ¼ inch thick

1 bunch kale, stems removed,
  coarsely torn into pieces

Briefly put the beef in the freezer to freeze partially in preparation for slicing thinly.

Mix the paprika, oregano, chili powder, garlic powder, black pepper, cayenne pepper, and dry mustard in a small container with a lid and set aside.

Thinly slice the beef across the grain into strips ⅛ inch thick. Sprinkle the strips liberally with the seasoning mix. (Save any leftover seasoning mix to use for other dishes.) Spray the bottom of a large skillet or stockpot with cooking spray and preheat over high heat. Add the meat and cook, stirring, for 5 minutes.

Add the potatoes, onions, broth, water, and garlic to the

skillet. The blackened spices will float to the top of the liquid as it heats. Cover and cook over medium heat for 20 minutes. Stir in the carrots and lay the kale on top. Cook, covered, until the carrots are tender, about 10 more minutes. Serve from the skillet or transfer to a large serving bowl. Serve with crusty bread for dunking.

Servings	Calories per serving	Fat (g)	Sodium (mg)
6 (2 cups each)	278	6	106

	Vegetables	Fruits/Juices	Dairy Foods	Grains
Food Group Serving(s):	4			

	Meat, Poultry, and Fish	Nuts, Seeds, and Legumes	Added Fats/Oils	Sweets
Food Group Serving(s):	1			

Chicken and Broccoli Bake

1 pound frozen chopped
  broccoli, thawed

1 cup finely chopped onions

1 clove fresh garlic, minced

¼ teaspoon freshly ground
  black pepper

1 cup cubed cooked white
  chicken meat without skin

1 (8-ounce) can sliced water
  chestnuts

½ cup fat-free sour cream

2 tablespoons skim milk

1 cup shredded low-fat
  mozzarella cheese

¼ cup grated Parmesan cheese

¾ teaspoon paprika

Place the broccoli in a baking dish with the onions, garlic, and pepper, spreading out the ingredients to cover the surface of the dish. Cover tightly and microwave on high until the vegetables are crisp-tender, about 3 to 4 minutes.

Arrange the chicken and water chestnuts evenly on top of the broccoli. Cover with wax paper and microwave on high for 3 minutes.

In a small mixing bowl, stir the sour cream and milk together; pour evenly over the contents of the baking dish. Sprinkle with the cheeses and paprika. Cover with wax paper again and microwave on medium-high (70%) until the cheeses are melted, 3 to 5 minutes.

Servings	Calories per serving	Fat (g)	Sodium (mg)
4 (1¼ cups each)	272	8	338

	Vegetables	Fruits/Juices	Dairy Foods	Grains
Food Group Serving(s):	2		1	

	Meat, Poultry, and Fish	Nuts, Seeds, and Legumes	Added Fats/Oils	Sweets
Food Group Serving(s):	0.5			

Chicken Fruity Stir-fry

———————⋀———————

1½ tablespoons sesame oil, divided

1¼ pounds boneless, skinless chicken breasts, cut into thin strips

½ cup sliced onions

1 cup carrot strips or slices

1 teaspoon dried basil

1 cup pea pods or snow peas

1 tablespoon water

¼ cup pine nuts

¼ cup chopped dried apricots

2 tablespoons raisins

1 large Golden Delicious apple, unpeeled, sliced

¾ cup Chinese duck sauce

Heat 1 tablespoon sesame oil in a skillet. Add the chicken and stir-fry until lightly browned and cooked through, about 4 minutes. Remove the chicken and keep warm. Heat the remaining oil in the skillet and stir-fry the onions, carrots, and basil until the carrots are tender.

Stir in the pea pods and water and stir-fry another 2 minutes. Stir in the pine nuts, apricots, and raisins.

Remove the skillet from the heat and stir in the apples. Return the chicken to the pan and stir to combine. Serve over hot cooked rice.

Top each serving with 2 tablespoons of duck sauce.

Servings	Calories per serving	Fat (g)	Sodium (mg)
5 (1 cup each) without rice	329	11	166

	Vegetables	Fruits/Juices	Dairy Foods	Grains
Food Group Serving(s):	0.5	1		
	Meat, Poultry, and Fish	Nuts, Seeds, and Legumes	Added Fats/Oils	Sweets
Food Group Serving(s):	0.5			

Chicken with Rice

———————/\———————

1⅓ cups chopped yellow
onions

1 cup chopped green bell
peppers

6 tablespoons safflower oil

1 cup low-sodium tomato
sauce

2 tablespoons chopped fresh
parsley

¼ teaspoon freshly ground
black pepper

1 tablespoon minced garlic

4 cups cooked long-grain
brown rice

14 ounces roasted skinless
chicken breast, cubed

In a large skillet, cook the onions and bell peppers in the oil
for about 5 minutes over medium heat. Combine the tomato
sauce with the parsley, pepper, and garlic, then stir into the
cooked vegetables. Stir in the rice and chicken, remove from
the heat, and serve warm.

Servings	Calories per serving	Fat (g)	Sodium (mg)
6 (1¼ cups each)	348	14	60

	Vegetables	Fruits/Juices	Dairy Foods	Grains
Food Group Serving(s):	1			1.5

	Meat, Poultry, and Fish	Nuts, Seeds, and Legumes	Added Fats/Oils	Sweets
Food Group Serving(s):	1			

Dave's Cajun Catfish

---/\\---

Seasoning Mix

4 tablespoons paprika

2 tablespoons dried oregano

2 teaspoons chili powder

1 teaspoon garlic powder

1 teaspoon freshly ground
    black pepper

½ teaspoon cayenne pepper

½ teaspoon dry mustard

Catfish

1 pound skinless catfish fillets

1 tablespoon vegetable oil

About ¼ teaspoon coarse salt

1 lemon, cut into wedges

Mix the spices together to make the seasoning mix. The mix can be stored in a covered container and used to season other dishes. This is the same seasoning used for Blackened Beef with Greens and Red Potatoes (pages 175–176), so it can be saved to make that recipe at another time.

Wash the catfish fillets and pat dry with paper towels. Liberally sprinkle seasoning mix onto both sides of the catfish (you will need about ½ of mix).

Heat the oil in a skillet over medium-high heat. Salt the catfish lightly, add to the skillet, and cook for 3 minutes. Turn and cook another 3 minutes or until the fish flakes easily. (Do not overcook.)

Serve with lemon wedges on the side.

Servings	Calories per serving	Fat (g)	Sodium (mg)
4 (4 ounces each)	216	14	228

	Vegetables	Fruits/Juices	Dairy Foods	Grains
Food Group Serving(s):				

	Meat, Poultry, and Fish	Nuts, Seeds, and Legumes	Added Fats/Oils	Sweets
Food Group Serving(s):	1			

Fettucine with Chicken and Vegetables

————————⋀————————

2 tablespoons olive oil
¼ cup lemon juice
¼ cup low-sodium chicken broth
2 teaspoons dried oregano
½ teaspoon ground cinnamon
1 pound boneless, skinless chicken breasts, cut into 1-inch cubes

4 cups cooked fettuccine (prepared from 1⅓ cups dried)
4½ cups cubed vegetables (any combination of bell peppers, broccoli, zucchini, carrots, spinach, and tomatoes)
½ cup fat-free sour cream
¼ cup grated Parmesan cheese

In a small bowl, combine the oil, lemon juice, chicken broth, oregano, and cinnamon. Pour over the chicken cubes and marinate 10 minutes.

Meanwhile, bring a large pot of water to a boil and cook the fettuccine until al dente, about 10 minutes for dried pasta or 2 to 3 minutes for fresh.

Drain the chicken, reserving the marinade. Lightly brown the chicken in a hot skillet over medium-high heat; add the vegetables and cook 3 to 5 minutes more. Pour in the marinade and simmer another 2 to 3 minutes.

Drain the pasta in a colander, rinse with hot water, and drain well again. Turn into a serving bowl and mix in the sour cream and Parmesan. Spoon the chicken and vegetables over the pasta and serve.

Servings	Calories per serving	Fat (g)	Sodium (mg)
6 (1⅔cups each)	432	8	247

	Vegetables	Fruits/Juices	Dairy Foods	Grains
Food Group Serving(s):	1			1

	Meat, Poultry, and Fish	Nuts, Seeds, and Legumes	Added Fats/Oils	Sweets
Food Group Serving(s):	0.5			

Grilled Tuna

—————⋀—————

2 cups peeled, seeded, and
diced tomatoes

1 tablespoon diced green
onions

1 clove garlic, minced

1 teaspoon lemon juice

1 tablespoon chopped fresh
cilantro

1½ pounds fresh yellowfin
tuna, cleaned and cut into
6 equal portions

Make a salsa by mixing together the tomatoes, green onions,
garlic, lemon juice, and cilantro.

Prepare an outdoor grill, letting the coals burn down until
covered with white ash. Grill the tuna for 6 to 8 minutes, then
turn and grill an additional 3 to 5 minutes, or longer for more
well done.

Serve the tuna on a platter, topped with the salsa.

Servings	Calories per serving	Fat (g)	Sodium (mg)
6 (3 ounces each)	177	6	50

	Vegetables	Fruits/Juices	Dairy Foods	Grains
Food Group Serving(s):	1			

	Meat, Poultry, and Fish	Nuts, Seeds, and Legumes	Added Fats/Oils	Sweets
Food Group Serving(s):	1			

Hawaiian Chicken Sandwich

———⋀———

1 (6-ounce) can pineapple
  slices in juice

¼ teaspoon dried oregano

¼ teaspoon garlic powder

4 (4-ounce) boneless, skinless
  chicken breast halves

¼ cup low-sodium light
  mayonnaise

1 (8-ounce) can water
  chestnuts, finely chopped

4 whole-wheat sandwich rolls

4 green bell peppers, seeded
  and cut into thin rings

12 lettuce leaves

Preheat the broiler or prepare an outdoor grill, letting the coals burn down until covered with white ash.

Put the pineapple with its juice, the oregano, and garlic powder in a shallow nonmetallic dish. Add the chicken to the dish, turn to coat on all sides, cover, and marinate 15 minutes in the refrigerator.

Grill or broil the chicken and pineapple, brushing with the reserved marinade, 5 to 8 minutes on each side or until the chicken is no longer pink in the center and the pineapple is golden brown. Discard any remaining marinade.

In a small bowl, combine the mayonnaise and water chestnuts and spread over the bottom of the rolls. Top with the chicken, pineapple, bell pepper rings, and lettuce. Cover with the top half of the rolls.

Servings	Calories per serving	Fat (g)	Sodium (mg)
4 (1 sandwich each)	413	8	464

	Vegetables	Fruits/Juices	Dairy Foods	Grains
Food Group Serving(s):	0.5	0.5		3

	Meat, Poultry, and Fish	Nuts, Seeds, and Legumes	Added Fats/Oils	Sweets
Food Group Serving(s):	1			

Mango and Black Bean Salad with Grilled Shrimp

——————⋀——————

Dressing

½ cup lime juice (from 3 medium limes)

1 tablespoon white wine vinegar

2 tablespoons Dijon mustard

2 cloves garlic, minced

2 teaspoons chili powder

2 teaspoons ground cumin

½ teaspoon freshly ground black pepper

2 tablespoons olive oil

Salad

3 (15-ounce) cans black beans, rinsed and drained

1 red bell pepper, seeded and chopped

1 ripe but firm mango, peeled and cut into ½-inch cubes

½ cup chopped fresh cilantro

¾ cup thinly sliced scallions, divided

3 cups torn greens (romaine and radicchio)

1 pound large or medium shrimp, shelled and deveined (optional)

Special equipment: If grilling shrimp, you will need wooden skewers. Soak the skewers in water before grilling to keep them from drying out.

To make the dressing, combine the lime juice, vinegar, mustard, garlic, chili powder, cumin, and pepper in a large mixing bowl. Whisk in the olive oil until well blended. Some of this dressing (about ¼ cup) can be used as a marinade for the grilled shrimp, if using.

To make the salad, add the beans, bell pepper, mango,

cilantro, and ½ cup of the scallions to the salad dressing in the large bowl and stir gently to combine. Refrigerate for 30 minutes to 1 hour before serving so that the salad is thoroughly chilled.

Just before serving, line a shallow bowl or platter with torn greens. Spoon the bean mixture over the greens and gently mix. Sprinkle with the remaining ¼ cup of scallions.

If using the shrimp, prepare an outdoor grill and let the coals burn down until covered with white ash. Toss the shrimp with the reserved ¼ cup of dressing and marinate for about 30 minutes. Thread the shrimp onto skewers and grill, turning once or twice, until lightly charred outside and no longer translucent within, about 6 minutes. Remove the skewers and top the salad with the shrimp.

Servings	Calories per serving	Fat (g)	Sodium (mg)
6 (1½ cups each)	244 without shrimp (319 with shrimp)	6 without shrimp (7 with shrimp)	143 without shrimp (314 with shrimp)

	Vegetables	Fruits/Juices	Dairy Foods	Grains
Food Group Serving(s):	1 (with or without shrimp)			

	Meat, Poultry, and Fish	Nuts, Seeds, and Legumes	Added Fats/Oils	Sweets
Food Group Serving(s):	1 (with shrimp)	1 (with or without shrimp)		

New Orleans Red Beans and Rice

———————⌄———————

1 cup dried red beans

1½ cups long-grain white rice

3 cups water

½ cup chopped onions

½ cup chopped celery

½ cup seeded and chopped
green bell pepper

2 cloves garlic, minced

1 (8-ounce) can unsalted
tomato sauce

1 teaspoon Worcestershire
sauce

2 teaspoons Cajun Spice Mix
(recipe below)

1 tablespoon light brown
sugar

½ teaspoon hot sauce, such as
Tabasco

¾ teaspoon salt

Cook the beans the day before, following the package directions or your usual procedure but with no salt. Drain and cool until ready to use.

Cook the rice in the water with no salt added until tender, about 20 minutes. While the rice is cooking, prepare the remaining ingredients.

Spray a medium stockpot with nonstick cooking spray and heat. Add the onions, celery, green pepper, and garlic and cook 2 to 3 minutes. Add the drained red beans, tomato sauce, Worcestershire sauce, Cajun Spice Mix, brown sugar, hot sauce, and salt. Lower the heat, cover, and simmer 15 minutes, stirring occasionally. Combine the bean mixture with the warm cooked rice and mix well.

Cajun Spice Mix: Mix together the following spices: ¼ cup paprika, 2 tablespoons dried oregano, 2 teaspoons chili powder, 1 teaspoon garlic powder, 1 teaspoon freshly ground black pepper, ½ teaspoon cayenne pepper, and ½ teaspoon dry mustard. This spice mix is used in several other DASH recipes.

Servings	Calories per serving	Fat (g)	Sodium (mg)
6 (1 cup each without rice)	194	1	544

	Vegetables	Fruits/Juices	Dairy Foods	Grains
Food Group Serving(s):	1			0.5

	Meat, Poultry, and Fish	Nuts, Seeds, and Legumes	Added Fats/Oils	Sweets
Food Group Serving(s):		1		

Northeast Gumbo

———— /\ ————

2 tablespoons canola oil

¼ cup thinly sliced green onions

1 yellow onion, finely chopped

1 medium red bell pepper, seeded and finely chopped

4 medium stalks celery, finely chopped

1 teaspoon garlic powder

¼ teaspoon cayenne pepper

¼ teaspoon salt

1 teaspoon dried thyme

2 cups low-sodium chicken broth

3 cups canned salt-free kidney beans

2 cups frozen spinach, thawed

1½ cups carrot strips or slices

1½ pounds boneless, skinless chicken breasts, cut into 1-inch cubes

½ cup minced fresh parsley

4 cups cooked rice

Heat the oil in a large saucepan over high heat. Add the green onions, yellow onion, bell pepper, and celery to the pan. Reduce the heat to medium and cook, stirring, until the vegetables are tender, about 3 minutes.

Add the garlic powder, cayenne, salt, and thyme and stir-fry for a few seconds. Add the broth and stir to combine. Raise the heat to high, bring the liquid to a boil, then add the beans, spinach, and carrots. Lower the heat, cover, and simmer for about 1 hour.

Add the chicken and parsley to the saucepan and simmer until the chicken is cooked through, about 15 minutes. Serve the gumbo over ⅔ cup rice per serving.

Servings	Calories per serving	Fat (g)	Sodium (mg)
6 (1 cup each)	361	12	289

	Vegetables	Fruits/Juices	Dairy Foods	Grains
Food Group Serving(s):	2			

	Meat, Poultry, and Fish	Nuts, Seeds, and Legumes	Added Fats/Oils	Sweets
Food Group Serving(s):	0.5	1.5		

Snapper with Greens

———————/\———————

1 pound red snapper fillets

¼ teaspoon freshly ground
black pepper

¾ cup plain low-fat yogurt

2 tablespoons low-sodium
light mayonnaise

2 tablespoons all-purpose
flour

2 tablespoons lemon juice

¼ teaspoon chopped fresh dill

2 bunches fresh spinach,
rinsed and drained but not
dried

½ teaspoon paprika

Preheat the oven to 350°F. Arrange the fish fillets in a single layer in a shallow 9 × 13-inch baking pan. Sprinkle with pepper.

In a mixing bowl, whisk together the yogurt, mayonnaise, flour, lemon juice, and dill. Spread the mixture over the fish using a spatula. Bake the fish, uncovered, until it flakes easily with a fork, about 20 to 30 minutes.

Meanwhile, put the wet spinach in a large skillet set over medium-high heat. Cover and cook, stirring occasionally, until the spinach wilts, about 2 to 3 minutes. Drain. To serve, arrange the spinach in a layer on a serving platter. Place the cooked fish on top. Spoon any extra sauce from the baking pan onto the fish and sprinkle with paprika.

Servings	Calories per serving	Fat (g)	Sodium (mg)
4 (4 ounces each)	215	4	277

	Vegetables	Fruits/Juices	Dairy Foods	Grains
Food Group Serving(s):	2			

	Meat, Poultry, and Fish	Nuts, Seeds, and Legumes	Added Fats/Oils	Sweets
Food Group Serving(s):	1			

Spicy Cod

————————∨————————

4 ounces cod fillets

1 teaspoon olive oil

1 teaspoon unsalted butter

1 teaspoon Spice Mixture
(recipe below)

Preheat the oven to 350°F. Put the fish in a baking dish and spread the oil, butter, and Spice Mixture evenly on top. Bake, uncovered, for about 15 minutes or until the fish just flakes with a fork. Serve over Scallion Rice (page 232).

Spice Mixture:

Mix the following spices ahead of time: 2 tablespoons ground white pepper, 2 tablespoons dried basil, 1⅓ tablespoons dried thyme, 1⅓ tablespoons onion powder, 3½ teaspoons garlic powder, 2 teaspoons freshly ground black pepper, and 1½ teaspoons cayenne pepper.

This spice mixture is good for other seafood and meat as well. It can even add flavor to some pasta dishes.

Servings	Calories per serving	Fat (g)	Sodium (mg)
1	344	11	111

	Vegetables	Fruits/Juices	Dairy Foods	Grains
Food Group Serving(s):				

	Meat, Poultry, and Fish	Nuts, Seeds, and Legumes	Added Fats/Oils	Sweets
Food Group Serving(s):	1			

Sweet-and-Sour Pork with Vegetables

½ cup blanched whole
  almonds

1 cup water

1½ pounds boneless top loin
  of pork, trimmed of all fat
  and cut into 1-inch cubes
  or strips

1 medium onion, sliced into
  half-moon-shaped slices

1 large green bell pepper,
  seeded and cut into 1-inch
  triangles

1 large tomato, roughly
  chopped

½ cup maple syrup

½ cup cider vinegar

½ cup low-sodium catsup

¼ cup reduced-sodium soy
  sauce

1 tablespoon cornstarch,
  dissolved in ½ cup water

1 cup canned pineapple
  chunks in juice, drained

6 cups cooked rice

Preheat the oven to 300°F.

Bake the almonds in the preheated oven for 15 minutes and set aside. Meanwhile, bring the water to a boil in a small saucepan. Add the pork and simmer for 5 minutes. Add the onion, bell pepper, and tomato to the pan and simmer for 5 additional minutes. Drain and reserve the pork and vegetables.

Put the maple syrup, vinegar, catsup, and soy sauce in a saucepan, bring to a boil over high heat, and boil for 2 minutes. Add the dissolved cornstarch and cook for 3 to 5 minutes to thicken. Then add the vegetables, pork, and pineapple chunks. Add the almonds, cook for 3 more minutes, and serve over cooked rice. Use 1 cup of rice for each serving of sweet-and-sour pork.

Servings	Calories per serving	Fat (g)	Sodium (mg)
6 (1 cup each without rice)	416	17	385

	Vegetables	Fruits/Juices	Dairy Foods	Grains
Food Group Serving(s):	1	0.5		

	Meat, Poultry, and Fish	Nuts, Seeds, and Legumes	Added Fats/Oils	Sweets
Food Group Serving(s):	0.5	0.5		

Swiss Cheese Sandwich

————/\————

2 teaspoons sunflower seeds

1 tablespoon low-sodium light mayonnaise

2 slices whole-wheat bread

4 raw spinach leaves

1 slice reduced-fat, reduced-sodium Swiss cheese

3 slices fresh tomato

2 slices red onion

1 green bell pepper ring

Mix the sunflower seeds into the mayonnaise and spread on the bread slices.

Build the sandwich by layering the ingredients on one slice of bread, then top with the other slice of bread.

Servings	Calories per serving	Fat (g)	Sodium (mg)
1	348	15	386

	Vegetables	Fruits/Juices	Dairy Foods	Grains
Food Group Serving(s):	3		0.5	2

	Meat, Poultry, and Fish	Nuts, Seeds, and Legumes	Added Fats/Oils	Sweets
Food Group Serving(s):				

Turkey Burger

—————⌄—————

3 ounces lean ground turkey

2 teaspoons prepared brown
mustard

2 slices whole-wheat bread or
1 whole-wheat sandwich
roll

4 raw spinach leaves

2 slices fresh tomato

1 slice red onion

Shape the turkey into a patty. Cook over medium heat in a
skillet coated with nonstick cooking spray.

Spread the mustard on the bread slices. Place the cooked
turkey patty on one slice, top with the remaining ingredients,
then top with the other slice of bread.

For a different presentation, crumble the turkey patty,
chop the vegetables, and serve in a whole-wheat pita pocket.

Servings	Calories per serving	Fat (g)	Sodium (mg)
1	305	10	542

	Vegetables	Fruits/Juices	Dairy Foods	Grains
Food Group Serving(s):	2.5			2

	Meat, Poultry, and Fish	Nuts, Seeds, and Legumes	Added Fats/Oils	Sweets
Food Group Serving(s):	0.5			

Vegetarian Lasagna

————————⋀————————

Sauce

½ cup chopped onions

3 cloves garlic, minced

¾ cup chopped green bell peppers

4½ cups chopped tomatoes

1½ cups water

1½ teaspoons crumbled bay leaf

¾ cup low-sodium tomato paste

Filling

¾ pound zucchini, thinly sliced

1 pound button mushrooms, thinly sliced

½ cup chopped onions

½ teaspoon dried rosemary

½ teaspoon dried oregano

½ cup 1% low-fat cottage cheese

½ cup shredded low-fat mozzarella cheese

4 egg whites

½ cup chopped fresh parsley

9 lasagna noodles, cooked

To prepare the sauce, coat a sauté pan with nonstick cooking spray. Add the onions, garlic, and peppers to the pan and sauté, stirring occasionally, until soft, about 2 minutes. Add the tomatoes with their liquid to the pan and simmer about 20 minutes, or until soft. Add the water, bay leaf, and tomato paste to the pan. Raise the heat, bring to a boil, then lower the heat and simmer about 45 minutes.

To prepare the filling, coat another sauté pan with nonstick cooking spray. Add the zucchini, mushrooms, and onions to the pan and cook, stirring occasionally, until soft, about 3 to 5 minutes. Add the rosemary and oregano to the pan. When the vegetables are tender, remove from the heat and set aside to cool. Add 2 cups of sauce to the vegetables. In a separate bowl, mix the cottage cheese, mozzarella, egg whites, and parsley.

Preheat the oven to 350°F.

Ladle 2 to 3 cups of sauce over the bottom of a 9 × 13-inch baking pan. Line with 3 lasagna noodles. Spread half of the cheese mixture over the pasta and top with half of the vegetable mixture. Repeat layering, beginning with sauce. Top with a layer of pasta and spread a small amount of sauce to cover it. Bake for about 1 hour in the preheated oven.

Servings	Calories per serving	Fat (g)	Sodium (mg)
9 (3 x 4 inch piece each)	187	2.5	149

	Vegetables	Fruits/Juices	Dairy Foods	Grains
Food Group Serving(s):	2		1	1

	Meat, Poultry, and Fish	Nuts, Seeds, and Legumes	Added Fats/Oils	Sweets
Food Group Serving(s):				

Vegetarian Spaghetti Sauce

———————⋁———————

2 small onions, chopped

3 cloves garlic

2 tablespoons olive oil

1 (8-ounce) can tomato sauce

1 (6-ounce) tomato paste

2 medium tomatoes, chopped

1¼ cups sliced zucchini

1 cup water

1 tablespoon dried oregano

1 tablespoon dried basil

Sauté the onions and garlic in the oil over medium heat for about 5 minutes. Add the tomato sauce, tomato paste, tomatoes, and zucchini. Stir the mixture, then add the water and herbs. Bring to a boil, then simmer for about 5 minutes. Serve over cooked spaghetti.

Servings	Calories per serving	Fat (g)	Sodium (mg)
7 (⅔cups each)	79	4	207

	Vegetables	Fruits/Juices	Dairy Foods	Grains
Food Group Serving(s):	0.5			

	Meat, Poultry, and Fish	Nuts, Seeds, and Legumes	Added Fats/Oils	Sweets
Food Group Serving(s):				

Vermont Roast with Brown Mustard

1½ pounds boneless, skinless chicken breasts, cut into 1-inch cubes

¾ cup maple syrup, divided

4 carrots, cut into large chunks

4 white onions, cut into large chunks

1 pound parsnips, cut into large chunks

3 sweet potatoes, cut into large chunks

¼ teaspoon freshly ground black pepper

¼ teaspoon dried thyme

1 tablespoon dried parsley flakes

1 cup low-sodium chicken broth

1 teaspoon paprika

Spicy brown mustard, for serving

Preheat the oven to 375°F. Combine the chicken cubes and ¼ cup of the maple syrup in a small bowl. Toss to combine, cover, and refrigerate until ready to use.

Spread the carrots, onions, parsnips, and sweet potatoes over the bottom of a 9 × 9-inch baking dish. Sprinkle the pepper, thyme, and parsley over the vegetables.

Pour the remaining ½ cup maple syrup evenly over the vegetables, then pour the chicken broth into the dish. Stir to distribute the ingredients evenly. Cover and bake in the preheated oven about 1½ hours. Every 20 minutes or so, stir the vegetables so that they remain moist.

Sprinkle the chicken with the paprika and stir to combine with the vegetables. Bake for another 20 minutes. Serve with spicy brown mustard for dipping.

Servings	Calories per serving	Fat (g)	Sodium (mg)
6 (2½ cups each)	477	11	143

	Vegetables	Fruits/Juices	Dairy Foods	Grains
Food Group Serving(s):	3			

	Meat, Poultry, and Fish	Nuts, Seeds, and Legumes	Added Fats/Oils	Sweets
Food Group Serving(s):	1			

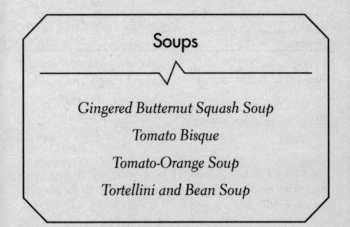

Soups

Gingered Butternut Squash Soup

Tomato Bisque

Tomato-Orange Soup

Tortellini and Bean Soup

Gingered Butternut Squash Soup

———————⌄———————

1 tablespoon canola oil

2 cloves garlic, minced

1 cup finely chopped onions

1 cup finely chopped celery

1½ tablespoons all-purpose flour

1 (14.5-ounce) can vegetable broth

2 cups water

2 cups 1-inch cubes butternut squash

1 cup finely chopped carrots

1 (19-ounce) can cannellini beans, drained, ½ cup liquid reserved

1 teaspoon grated fresh ginger

1½ teaspoons curry powder

1 (8-ounce) container plain low-fat yogurt, for topping

¼ cup finely sliced green onions, for topping

Heat the oil in a large soup pot over medium-high heat. Add the garlic, onions, and celery to the pot and sauté for about 5 minutes. Add the flour and stir to blend. Slowly add the vegetable broth and water to the pot, stirring to blend. Add the squash, carrots, beans, and reserved bean liquid. Simmer for 15 minutes or until tender. Remove 2 cups, puree in a blender until smooth, and stir back into the soup to thicken. Simmer for 15 minutes. Add the ginger and curry powder and simmer for an additional 15 minutes.

Garnish each serving with a dollop of yogurt and a sprinkling of green onions.

Servings	Calories per serving	Fat (g)	Sodium (mg)
4 (1½ cups each)	268	6	415

	Vegetables	Fruits/Juices	Dairy Foods	Grains
Food Group Serving(s):	1.5			

	Meat, Poultry, and Fish	Nuts, Seeds, and Legumes	Added Fats/Oils	Sweets
Food Group Serving(s):		1.5		

Tomato Bisque

¾ teaspoon olive oil

3½ cups chopped onions

½ cup chopped celery

1 teaspoon fresh or dried tarragon

¼ teaspoon fresh or dried thyme

¼ cup long-grain white rice

3 pounds plum tomatoes, seeded and roughly chopped

5 cups low-sodium chicken broth

½ cup low-sodium tomato paste

1 small bay leaf

½ cup lightly packed fresh basil leaves

¼ teaspoon coarse salt

¼ teaspoon freshly ground black pepper

Heat the oil in a soup pot over medium-high heat. Add the onions and celery to the pot and sauté, stirring occasionally, for 3 minutes. Add the tarragon, thyme, rice, tomatoes, and broth to the pot. Raise the heat to high, bring to a boil, then add the tomato paste and bay leaf. Lower the heat and simmer for 30 minutes or until the vegetables are crisp-tender. Add the basil, salt, and pepper.

Remove the bay leaf and puree the soup in a blender until the desired consistency is reached. (You may need to do this in batches.)

Reheat the soup and serve.

Servings	Calories per serving	Fat (g)	Sodium (mg)
10 (1 cup each)	98	2	120

	Vegetables	Fruits/Juices	Dairy Foods	Grains
Food Group Serving(s):	1			

	Meat, Poultry, and Fish	Nuts, Seeds, and Legumes	Added Fats/Oils	Sweets
Food Group Serving(s):				

Tomato-Orange Soup

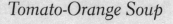

1 teaspoon olive oil

3 cups roughly chopped
   white onions

3 (28-ounce) cans whole
   peeled tomatoes

Grated zest of 2 oranges,
   divided

1 cup fresh orange juice

1 teaspoon coarse salt

½ teaspoon freshly ground
   black pepper

¼ teaspoon ground cloves

2 tablespoons chopped fresh
   basil

In a heavy-bottomed soup pot, heat the oil over medium-high
heat. Add the onions to the pot and sauté, stirring occasionally, until translucent, about 3 minutes. Add the tomatoes and
their liquid, raise the heat to high, and bring to a boil. Lower
the heat and simmer for 45 minutes. Remove from the heat
and stir in all but 2 tablespoons of the orange zest, the orange
juice, salt, pepper, and cloves. Let the soup cool, then puree
in a blender. (You may need to do this in batches.) Serve
chilled with a garnish of basil and orange zest.

Servings	Calories per serving	Fat (g)	Sodium (mg)
10 (1 cup each)	77	1	261

	Vegetables	Fruits/Juices	Dairy Foods	Grains
Food Group Serving(s):	1			

	Meat, Poultry, and Fish	Nuts, Seeds, and Legumes	Added Fats/Oils	Sweets
Food Group Serving(s):				

Tortellini and Bean Soup

———————⋁———————

1 teaspoon olive oil

2 cups roughly chopped white onions

1 small red bell pepper, seeded and roughly chopped

3 cloves garlic, minced

1 teaspoon Italian seasoning

⅔ cup water

2 cups roughly chopped raw spinach

1 (16-ounce) can no-salt-added navy beans, drained

1 (14.5-ounce) can low-sodium chicken broth

1 (14.5-ounce) can no-salt-added whole tomatoes

1 (14-ounce) can artichoke hearts packed in water, drained

9 ounces cheese tortellini

Heat the oil in a soup pot over medium-high heat. Add the onions, bell pepper, garlic, and Italian seasoning to the pot. Sauté, stirring occasionally, for 5 minutes or until the ingredients are tender. Add the water, spinach, beans, broth, tomatoes with their juice, and artichokes to the pot. Raise the heat to high and bring to a boil. Lower the heat and simmer for 2 minutes. Add the tortellini to the pot and cook until thoroughly heated, about 7 minutes. Serve.

Servings	Calories per serving	Fat (g)	Sodium (mg)
6 (1½ cups each)	263	5	194

	Vegetables	Fruits/Juices	Dairy Foods	Grains
Food Group Serving(s):	2		0.5	0.5

	Meat, Poultry, and Fish	Nuts, Seeds, and Legumes	Added Fats/Oils	Sweets
Food Group Serving(s):		1		

Vegetable Side Dishes

Broccoli Rabe

Green Beans with Almonds

Kale with Sesame Seeds

Limas and Spinach

Molasses-Braised Collards

Sautéed Collard Greens

Stuffed Acorn Squash

Sweet-Potato Chips

Broccoli Rabe

———————⌄———————

2 pounds broccoli rabe (rapini),
    separated into stalks
1 cup low-sodium chicken broth

In a pot large enough to hold the broccoli rabe, bring water to
a boil over high heat. Place the broccoli rabe in a steamer basket and lower into the boiling water. Cook for about 5 minutes
to cut the bitterness and bring out the brilliant color. An alternative to steaming is to cook in a microwave until tender.

Meanwhile, bring the chicken broth to a boil in a 2-quart
saucepan over high heat, then lower the heat to simmer the
broth. Remove the broccoli rabe from the steamer basket and
simmer in the chicken broth until just tender.

Servings	Calories per serving	Fat (g)	Sodium (mg)
4 (1½ cups each)	48	0.5	67

	Vegetables	Fruits/Juices	Dairy Foods	Grains
Food Group Serving(s):	2.5			

	Meat, Poultry, and Fish	Nuts, Seeds, and Legumes	Added Fats/Oils	Sweets
Food Group Serving(s):				

Green Beans with Almonds

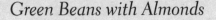

1 pound frozen green beans
2 teaspoons olive oil

¼ cup blanched slivered almonds
¼ teaspoon lemon pepper

Steam or microwave the frozen beans according to package directions. Meanwhile, heat the olive oil in a sauté pan over medium heat. Add the almonds to the pan and cook, stirring occasionally, until heated, about 2 minutes. Transfer the almonds to a stainless steel mixing bowl. Toss with the lemon pepper. Add the beans to the bowl and toss again. Serve immediately.

Servings	Calories per serving	Fat (g)	Sodium (mg)
6 (1½ cups each)	72	5	20

	Vegetables	Fruits/Juices	Dairy Foods	Grains
Food Group Serving(s):	1			

	Meat, Poultry, and Fish	Nuts, Seeds, and Legumes	Added Fats/Oils	Sweets
Food Group Serving(s):				

Kale with Sesame Seeds

———————⌄———————

¼ cup sesame seeds

1 pound kale, stems removed,
   coarsely torn into pieces

½ tablespoon sesame oil

1 slice gingerroot

1 clove garlic, minced

2 tablespoons balsamic
   vinegar

Toast the sesame seeds in a dry skillet over medium heat until they color and start to pop, about 2 minutes. Transfer the seeds to a sheet of waxed paper. Cover with another sheet of waxed paper and use a rolling pin to crush them. Set aside.

Bring a small pot of water to a boil over high heat. Place the kale in a steamer basket and lower into the pot of boiling water for 2 minutes to cut the bitterness and bring out the brilliant color, or cook in a microwave until tender. Drain and reserve.

Heat the sesame oil in a 2-quart sauté pan over medium heat. Add the ginger and garlic and sauté for about 2 minutes. Add the kale and stir to coat. Cover and cook for 3 to 5 minutes or until the kale is soft. Top with the toasted sesame seeds. Place in a serving bowl and add the balsamic vinegar.

Servings	Calories per serving	Fat (g)	Sodium (mg)
4 (¾ cup each)	117	4	53

	Vegetables	Fruits/Juices	Dairy Foods	Grains
Food Group Serving(s):	1.5			

	Meat, Poultry, and Fish	Nuts, Seeds, and Legumes	Added Fats/Oils	Sweets
Food Group Serving(s):				

Limas and Spinach

———————/\———————

2 cups frozen lima beans,
    thawed

1 tablespoon vegetable oil

½ cup roughly chopped
    onions

1 cup fennel strips, about
    1 × 1½ inches

¼ cup low-sodium chicken
    broth

4 cups tightly packed fresh
    spinach

1 tablespoon red wine vinegar

⅛ teaspoon freshly ground
    black pepper

1 tablespoon minced fresh
    chives

Steam or boil the lima beans for about 10 minutes, or cook in
a microwave according to package directions. Drain.

Heat the oil in a skillet over medium heat. Add the onions
and fennel and cook, stirring occasionally, for 5 to 10 minutes. Add the lima beans and broth to the skillet, cover, and
cook for 2 minutes. Stir in the spinach. Cover and cook until
the spinach has wilted, about 2 minutes. Stir in the vinegar
and pepper. Remove from the heat, cover, and let stand for 30
seconds.

Sprinkle with chives and serve.

Servings	Calories per serving	Fat (g)	Sodium (mg)
7 (¾ cup each)	80	2	110

	Vegetables	Fruits/Juices	Dairy Foods	Grains
Food Group Serving(s):	1.5			

	Meat, Poultry, and Fish	Nuts, Seeds, and Legumes	Added Fats/Oils	Sweets
Food Group Serving(s):				

Molasses-Braised Collards

———⌄———

¼ cup water

2 tablespoons light molasses

2 teaspoons hot sauce, such as
    Tabasco

1 tablespoon canola oil

2 cups thinly sliced onions

2 cloves garlic, minced

1¾ pounds collard greens,
    coarsely chopped

¼ teaspoon freshly ground
    black pepper

In a small bowl, mix together the water, molasses, and hot sauce.

In a large skillet, heat the oil over medium heat. Add the onions and garlic and cook, stirring, until golden, about 10 minutes. Stir the collards into the contents of the skillet. (You may need to cook some of the collards down before adding all.) Add the molasses mixture and stir gently. Lower the heat and cook, covered, for 40 minutes, stirring occasionally. Season with pepper.

Servings	Calories per serving	Fat (g)	Sodium (mg)
4 (1 cup each)	141	4	52

	Vegetables	Fruits/Juices	Dairy Foods	Grains
Food Group Serving(s):	2			

	Meat, Poultry, and Fish	Nuts, Seeds, and Legumes	Added Fats/Oils	Sweets
Food Group Serving(s):				

Sautéed Collard Greens

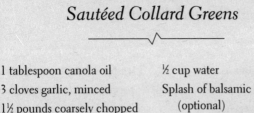

1 tablespoon canola oil

3 cloves garlic, minced

1½ pounds coarsely chopped
    collard greens, stems and
    large veins removed

½ cup water

Splash of balsamic vinegar
    (optional)

Freshly ground black pepper
    to taste (optional)

Heat the oil in a wide sauté pan over medium heat. Add the
garlic, stir, and add the collards (you may have to add the collards in batches to allow some to wilt before all will fit in the
pan). Add the water and stir occasionally until the collards are
bright green and tender. If desired, add a splash of balsamic
vinegar and pepper to taste.

Servings	Calories per serving	Fat (g)	Sodium (mg)
4 (1 cup each)	84	4	35

	Vegetables	Fruits/Juices	Dairy Foods	Grains
Food Group Serving(s):	2			

	Meat, Poultry, and Fish	Nuts, Seeds, and Legumes	Added Fats/Oils	Sweets
Food Group Serving(s):				

Stuffed Acorn Squash

———⌄———

1 pound acorn squash	1 teaspoon light brown sugar
¼ cup water	½ teaspoon ground cinnamon
½ cup unsweetened applesauce	

Cut the squash in half lengthwise, scoop out the seeds, and place the halves, cut side down, in a casserole dish. Pour the water around the squash and cover the casserole tightly with a lid or plastic wrap. Microwave on high for 10 minutes. Meanwhile, in a small bowl, combine the applesauce, brown sugar, and cinnamon.

Remove the cover, turn the squash cut side up, and divide the applesauce mixture between the centers. Microwave, uncovered, for an additional 5 minutes or until the squash is tender. The squash can be served as is or scooped out and served in a bowl.

Servings	Calories per serving	Fat (g)	Sodium (mg)
2 (¾ cup each)	103		8

	Vegetables	Fruits/Juices	Dairy Foods	Grains
Food Group Serving(s):	1.5	0.5		

	Meat, Poultry, and Fish	Nuts, Seeds, and Legumes	Added Fats/Oils	Sweets
Food Group Serving(s):				

Sweet-Potato Chips

———————/\/———————

1 medium sweet potato

Preheat the oven to 350°F.

Cut the sweet potato into very thin slices. Spray a sheet pan with nonstick cooking spray. Lay the sweet potato slices on the sheet pan and spray the top of the slices with cooking spray. Bake for about 25 to 35 minutes or until lightly browned. Cooled at room temperature, the sweet-potato chips will turn crispy.

Servings	Calories per serving	Fat (g)	Sodium (mg)
1	103		8

	Vegetables	Fruits/Juices	Dairy Foods	Grains
Food Group Serving(s):	2			

	Meat, Poultry, and Fish	Nuts, Seeds, and Legumes	Added Fats/Oils	Sweets
Food Group Serving(s):				

Grains

Apple Cobbler

Blueberry Pancakes

Bulgur Wheat with Tomatoes

Couscous with Broccoli

Scallion Rice

Wild Rice Pilaf

Apple Cobbler

⌄

8 medium tart apples

1 large lemon (juice and
grated zest)

¾ cup brown sugar

2 cups old-fashioned oats

1 cup chopped dried fruit

1 teaspoon ground cinnamon

½ cup water

Preheat the oven to 325°F.

Core, peel, and slice the apples and place in a 4-quart baking dish or slow cooker. Squeeze the juice and grate the zest (about 2 tablespoons) from the lemon and add to the apples. Add the brown sugar, oats, dried fruit, cinnamon, and enough water to moisten (about ½ cup). Stir, mixing all the ingredients together. Bake for about 2 hours in the preheated oven or on high if using a slow cooker.

Shortcut: Use 1 quart of applesauce instead of the apples. Reduce the sugar to ½ cup. Cook until heated through.

Servings	Calories per serving	Fat (g)	Sodium (mg)
12 (1 cup each)	170	1	7

	Vegetables	Fruits/Juices	Dairy Foods	Grains
Food Group Serving(s):		1		1

	Meat, Poultry, and Fish	Nuts, Seeds, and Legumes	Added Fats/Oils	Sweets
Food Group Serving(s):				

Blueberry Pancakes

——————⋀——————

1 cup all-purpose flour	1½ cups buttermilk
½ cup whole-wheat flour	1 large egg
1 tablespoon granulated sugar	2 tablespoons water
1 teaspoon baking powder	¼ cup nonfat dry milk
½ teaspoon baking soda	1 cup blueberries

Separately mix the dry and wet ingredients except the blueberries. Combine the dry and wet ingredients, leaving the mixture somewhat lumpy. Stir in the blueberries or add to each pancake while cooking. Pour about ⅓ cup of batter for each pancake into a nonstick skillet and cook for 2 minutes on each side. Serve warm.

Servings	Calories per serving	Fat (g)	Sodium (mg)
10 (1 pancake each)	118	1	141

	Vegétables	Fruits/Juices	Dairy Foods	Grains
Food Group Serving(s):				1

	Meat, Poultry, and Fish	Nuts, Seeds, and Legumes	Added Fats/Oils	Sweets
Food Group Serving(s):				

Bulgur Wheat with Tomatoes

————————⋀————————

1 tablespoon olive oil

1 medium onion, finely chopped

1 medium green bell pepper, seeded and diced

4 medium plum tomatoes, roughly chopped

½ teaspoon ground cinnamon

½ teaspoon ground cumin

1 cup bulgur wheat

¼ cup raisins

1¾ cups low-sodium chicken broth

¾ cup water

⅛ teaspoon freshly ground black pepper

2 tablespoons chopped fresh parsley

In a 3-quart saucepan, heat the oil over medium heat. Add the onion and green bell pepper to the pan and cook, stirring occasionally, until the onion is translucent, about 3 minutes. Add the tomatoes, cinnamon, cumin, bulgur wheat, and raisins to the pan. Add the broth and water, raise the heat to high, and bring to a boil. Lower the heat until the liquid is simmering. Cook, covered, until the bulgur wheat is tender, 15 to 20 minutes. Stir in the pepper and parsley and serve hot.

Servings	Calories per serving	Fat (g)	Sodium (mg)
5 (1 cup each)	183	4	52

	Vegetables	Fruits/Juices	Dairy Foods	Grains
Food Group Serving(s):	1.5			1

	Meat, Poultry, and Fish	Nuts, Seeds, and Legumes	Added Fats/Oils	Sweets
Food Group Serving(s):				

Couscous with Broccoli

―――――――∧―――――――

2 medium plum tomatoes,
  roughly chopped

¼ cup roughly chopped green
  onions

¼ cup raisins

¼ teaspoon dried basil

¼ teaspoon ground cumin

¼ teaspoon freshly ground
  black pepper

1 tablespoon olive oil

2 cups water

2½ cups broccoli florets

1¾ cups couscous

In a mixing bowl, combine the tomatoes with the green onions, raisins, basil, cumin, pepper, and olive oil. Set aside. Place the water and broccoli florets in a large saucepan and bring to boil over high heat. Lower the heat to medium and add the tomato mixture to the saucepan, then stir in the couscous. Cover and remove from the heat. Let stand for 5 minutes. Fluff lightly with a fork before serving.

Servings	Calories per serving	Fat (g)	Sodium (mg)
6 (¾ cup each)	242	3	23

	Vegetables	Fruits/Juices	Dairy Foods	Grains
Food Group Serving(s):	1			0.5

	Meat, Poultry, and Fish	Nuts, Seeds, and Legumes	Added Fats/Oils	Sweets
Food Group Serving(s):				

Scallion Rice

———————⌄———————

1 cup cooked brown rice
1 tablespoon chopped green
   onions (scallions)

Mix the cooked rice with the chopped scallions. Serve with Spicy Cod (page 197) or another dish of your choice.

Servings	Calories per serving	Fat (g)	Sodium (mg)
1	248	2	13

	Vegetables	Fruits/Juices	Dairy Foods	Grains
Food Group Serving(s):				2

	Meat, Poultry, and Fish	Nuts, Seeds, and Legumes	Added Fats/Oils	Sweets
Food Group Serving(s):				

Wild Rice Pilaf

½ cup wild rice

½ cup long-grain white rice, preferably basmati

3 cups fat-free, low-sodium chicken broth

½ cup chopped pecans

1 cup golden raisins

1 tablespoon olive oil

⅓ cup fresh orange juice

¼ cup chopped fresh mint, plus a few sprigs for garnish

¼ cup thinly sliced green onions

½ teaspoon salt

Freshly ground black pepper to taste

1 tablespoon grated orange zest (from 1 large orange)

Rinse the wild rice in a strainer under cold water. Place the wild rice and white rice in a medium saucepan. Add the broth and bring to a rolling boil over high heat. Lower the heat and simmer gently for 25 minutes, uncovered. Check for tenderness.

Meanwhile, heat the pecans in a small, heavy skillet over medium-high heat. Watch closely so they do not burn. Toast until lightly browned, about 8 minutes.

Transfer the rice to a serving bowl. Add the pecans and raisins.

In a small bowl, combine the oil, orange juice, chopped mint, green onions, salt, and pepper. Pour over the rice mixture and toss gently. Let stand for about 2 hours to allow the flavors to mix. Serve at room temperature or warm in a microwave. Garnish with mint sprigs and orange zest. This dish is also good cold as a salad.

Servings	Calories per serving	Fat (g)	Sodium (mg)
8 (⅔ cup each)	222	7	237

	Vegetables	Fruits/Juices	Dairy Foods	Grains
Food Group Serving(s):				1

	Meat, Poultry, and Fish	Nuts, Seeds, and Legumes	Added Fats/Oils	Sweets
Food Group Serving(s):				

Salads

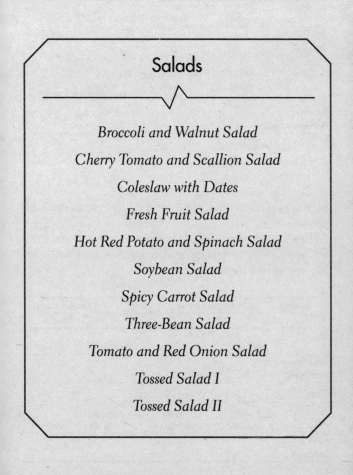

Broccoli and Walnut Salad

Cherry Tomato and Scallion Salad

Coleslaw with Dates

Fresh Fruit Salad

Hot Red Potato and Spinach Salad

Soybean Salad

Spicy Carrot Salad

Three-Bean Salad

Tomato and Red Onion Salad

Tossed Salad I

Tossed Salad II

Broccoli and Walnut Salad

————————/\————————

3 cups roughly chopped
broccoli florets

½ medium head cauliflower,
roughly chopped

1 cup raisins

¾ cup chopped onions

1 small red bell pepper,
seeded and thinly sliced

½ cup chopped walnuts

¼ cup red wine vinegar

¼ cup olive oil

6 to 12 large lettuce leaves

2 beefsteak tomatoes, cut into
wedges

In a large mixing bowl, combine the broccoli, cauliflower, raisins, onions, bell pepper, and walnuts.

In a separate bowl, whisk together the vinegar and olive oil. Toss with the combined salad ingredients and serve on lettuce leaves with tomato wedges.

Servings	Calories per serving	Fat (g)	Sodium (mg)
6 (1⅓ cup each)	257	15	33

	Vegetables	Fruits/Juices	Dairy Foods	Grains
Food Group Serving(s):	1.5	0.5		

	Meat, Poultry, and Fish	Nuts, Seeds, and Legumes	Added Fats/Oils	Sweets
Food Group Serving(s):				

Cherry Tomato and Scallion Salad

―――――――⌄―――――――

2 pints cherry tomatoes,
    halved
½ cup thinly sliced green
    onions (scallions)

¼ cup chopped fresh parsley
1 tablespoon balsamic vinegar
1 tablespoon olive oil

In a large bowl, combine the tomatoes and scallions. Sprinkle with the parsley.

In a small bowl, whisk together the vinegar and oil. Pour the dressing over the salad and toss again.

Servings	Calories per serving	Fat (g)	Sodium (mg)
4 (1 cup each)	64	4	14

	Vegetables	Fruits/Juices	Dairy Foods	Grains
Food Group Serving(s):	2			

	Meat, Poultry, and Fish	Nuts, Seeds, and Legumes	Added Fats/Oils	Sweets
Food Group Serving(s):				

Coleslaw with Dates

_____⌄_____

1½ cups shredded green
　cabbage
1½ cups shredded red cabbage
½ cup chopped pitted dates
2 tablespoons olive oil
2 tablespoons balsamic
　vinegar

1 teaspoon honey
¼ teaspoon freshly ground
　black pepper
2 tablespoons blanched
　slivered almonds

In a large salad bowl, combine the cabbages and dates.

In a small bowl, whisk together the oil, vinegar, honey, and pepper. Pour the dressing over the coleslaw, toss lightly, then sprinkle with almonds and toss again.

Servings	Calories per serving	Fat (g)	Sodium (mg)
8 (⅓ cup each)	85	5	6

	Vegetables	Fruits/Juices	Dairy Foods	Grains
Food Group Serving(s):	0.5	0.5		

	Meat, Poultry, and Fish	Nuts, Seeds, and Legumes	Added Fats/Oils	Sweets
Food Group Serving(s):				

Fresh Fruit Salad

---/\---

2 cups hulled and halved
   fresh strawberries

1 cantaloupe, cut into 1-inch
   chunks

2 medium bananas, sliced
   into bite-size pieces

Place all the ingredients in a serving bowl. Gently toss
and serve.

Servings	Calories per serving	Fat (g)	Sodium (mg)
4 (1½ cups each)	127	1	26

	Vegetables	Fruits/Juices	Dairy Foods	Grains
Food Group Serving(s):		2.5		

	Meat, Poultry, and Fish	Nuts, Seeds, and Legumes	Added Fats/Oils	Sweets
Food Group Serving(s):				

Hot Red Potato and Spinach Salad

———————√———————

1 pound red potatoes, cut into small pieces (about 2 cups)

1 bunch fresh spinach, stems removed, roughly chopped

1 tablespoon olive oil

2 cloves garlic, minced

½ red onion, cut into thin slices

1½ teaspoons dried rosemary

1 (15-ounce) can kidney beans, rinsed and drained

2 tablespoons balsamic vinegar

2 tablespoons lemon juice

¼ teaspoon coarse salt

¼ teaspoon freshly ground black pepper

2 tablespoons grated Parmesan cheese

Set a pot of water over high heat and bring to a boil. Place the potatoes in a steamer basket, lower into the pot, and steam until tender, about 20 minutes. Drain. (Potatoes can also be microwaved; follow microwave instructions.) Place the spinach in a large serving bowl and set aside.

Heat the olive oil in a large skillet and add the garlic, onion, and rosemary. Cook, stirring occasionally, until the onion is translucent, about 5 minutes. Add the potatoes, beans, vinegar, lemon juice, salt, and pepper to the skillet. Raise the heat and continue to cook until the liquid boils.

Pour the hot vegetable mixture over the spinach leaves and toss until the spinach is coated. Top with Parmesan cheese. Serve hot.

Servings	Calories per serving	Fat (g)	Sodium (mg)
8 (1½ cups each)	114	2.5	277

	Vegetables	Fruits/Juices	Dairy Foods	Grains
Food Group Serving(s):	2			

	Meat, Poultry, and Fish	Nuts, Seeds, and Legumes	Added Fats/Oils	Sweets
Food Group Serving(s):		0.5		

Soybean Salad

———⌄———

1 (15-ounce) can no-salt-added soybeans, rinsed and drained

1 (15-ounce) can low-salt black beans, rinsed and drained

1 large green bell pepper, seeded and roughly chopped

½ medium red onion, roughly chopped

½ cup roughly chopped fresh parsley

2 tablespoons olive oil

2 tablespoons red wine vinegar

⅛ teaspoon freshly ground black pepper

In a salad bowl, combine the soybeans, black beans, bell pepper, onion, and parsley.

In a separate bowl, whisk together the oil, vinegar, and pepper. Drizzle over the salad and toss gently.

Servings	Calories per serving	Fat (g)	Sodium (mg)
6 (¾ cup each)	141	5	149

	Vegetables	Fruits/Juices	Dairy Foods	Grains
Food Group Serving(s):	0.5			

	Meat, Poultry, and Fish	Nuts, Seeds, and Legumes	Added Fats/Oils	Sweets
Food Group Serving(s):		1.5		

Spicy Carrot Salad

6 medium carrots, cut into
    julienne strips or coarsely
    grated
½ cup finely chopped shallots
1½ tablespoons granulated
    sugar
⅛ teaspoon salt
¼ teaspoon chopped fresh
    basil

⅛ teaspoon ground cumin
¼ teaspoon freshly ground
    black pepper
pinch of cayenne pepper
    (optional)
3 tablespoons lemon juice
½ cup minced fresh parsley

Place the carrots and shallots in a serving bowl.

In a small bowl, combine the sugar, salt, basil, and cumin. Toss this mixture with the carrots and shallots. Season with black pepper and cayenne, if desired.

Add the lemon juice and toss. Marinate at room temperature for 1 hour. Sprinkle with the parsley and serve at room temperature.

Servings	Calories per serving	Fat (g)	Sodium (mg)
4 (1 cup each)	91		141

	Vegetables	Fruits/Juices	Dairy Foods	Grains
Food Group Serving(s):	2			

	Meat, Poultry, and Fish	Nuts, Seeds, and Legumes	Added Fats/Oils	Sweets
Food Group Serving(s):				

Three-Bean Salad

$$\diagdown$$

Salad

½ cup finely chopped red
  onions

½ cup finely chopped green
  onions

¼ cup finely chopped fresh
  parsley

1 (15-ounce) can kidney
  beans, rinsed and drained

¾ pound fresh green beans or
  thawed frozen beans

¾ pound fresh yellow wax
  beans or thawed frozen
  beans

Dressing

2 tablespoons olive oil

3 tablespoons red wine
  vinegar

1 tablespoon lemon juice

¼ teaspoon freshly ground
  black pepper

Place all the salad ingredients in a serving bowl.

In a separate bowl, whisk together the dressing ingredients. Drizzle the dressing over the salad and toss.

Servings	Calories per serving	Fat (g)	Sodium (mg)
6 (1 cup each)	323	5	199

	Vegetables	Fruits/Juices	Dairy Foods	Grains
Food Group Serving(s):	0.5			

	Meat, Poultry, and Fish	Nuts, Seeds, and Legumes	Added Fats/Oils	Sweets
Food Group Serving(s):		1.5		

Tomato and Red Onion Salad

———————⋀———————

3 tablespoons red wine
vinegar

1 tablespoon olive oil

¼ teaspoon freshly ground
black pepper

4 ripe tomatoes, each cut into
4 wedges

½ cup thinly sliced red onions

½ cucumber, thinly sliced

⅓ cup lightly packed roughly
chopped fresh basil

2 cups mixed salad greens

In a small bowl, whisk together the vinegar, oil, and pepper.

Place the tomatoes, onions, cucumber, and basil in a large
serving bowl. Drizzle the dressing over the salad and gently
toss. Let stand at least 1 hour before serving. Serve over a bed
of mixed salad greens.

Servings	Calories per serving	Fat (g)	Sodium (mg)
4 (1½ cups each)	96	4	20

	Vegetables	Fruits/Juices	Dairy Foods	Grains
Food Group Serving(s):	2.5			

	Meat, Poultry, and Fish	Nuts, Seeds, and Legumes	Added Fats/Oils	Sweets
Food Group Serving(s):				

Tossed Salad I

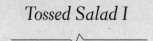

¾ cup mixed salad greens
¼ cup cherry tomatoes
1 tablespoon balsamic vinegar

Place all the ingredients in a small bowl and gently toss to distribute the balsamic vinegar.

Servings	Calories per serving	Fat (g)	Sodium (mg)
1 (1 cup each)	25		18

	Vegetables	Fruits/Juices	Dairy Foods	Grains
Food Group Serving(s):	1.5			

	Meat, Poultry, and Fish	Nuts, Seeds, and Legumes	Added Fats/Oils	Sweets
Food Group Serving(s):				

Tossed Salad II

———————⌄———————

1 cup mixed salad greens

¼ small green bell pepper,
    seeded and thinly sliced

2 wedges fresh tomato

⅓ red onion, chopped

3 cucumber slices

1 teaspoon olive oil

1 tablespoon balsamic vinegar

Place all the ingredients in a small bowl and gently toss.

Servings	Calories per serving	Fat (g)	Sodium (mg)
1 (2½ cups)	117	5.5	42

	Vegetables	Fruits/Juices	Dairy Foods	Grains
Food Group Serving(s):	3.5			

	Meat, Poultry, and Fish	Nuts, Seeds, and Legumes	Added Fats/Oils	Sweets
Food Group Serving(s):			1	

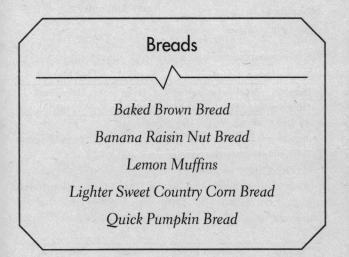

Breads

Baked Brown Bread

Banana Raisin Nut Bread

Lemon Muffins

Lighter Sweet Country Corn Bread

Quick Pumpkin Bread

Baked Brown Bread

———————⋁———————

½ cup all-purpose flour
½ cup rye flour
½ cup yellow cornmeal
2 teaspoons baking soda
½ cup light molasses

½ cup raisins, parboiled until plump
¾ cup plain nonfat yogurt
¾ cup skim milk

In a small bowl, mix the flours, cornmeal, and baking soda together.

In a separate bowl, beat together the molasses, raisins, yogurt, and milk. Stir in the dry ingredients.

Spray a 5 × 9-inch loaf pan with nonstick cooking spray. Pour the batter into the pan and let stand for 1 hour.

Preheat the oven to 350°F.

Bake the loaf for about 1 hour or until a toothpick inserted into the center comes out clean. This tastes so good that the remaining bread can be used another day for dessert.

Servings	Calories per serving	Fat (g)	Sodium (mg)
10 (¾-inch-thick slice each)	147	0.5	284

	Vegetables	Fruits/Juices	Dairy Foods	Grains
Food Group Servings(s):				1

	Meat, Poultry, and Fish	Nuts, Seeds, and Legumes	Added Fats/Oils	Sweets
Food Group Servings(s):				

Banana Raisin Nut Bread

—————⋀—————

½ cup vanilla low-fat yogurt

½ cup firmly packed light brown sugar

½ cup egg substitute or 4 egg whites

4 teaspoons lemon juice

2 tablespoons vegetable oil

1 cup mashed bananas (from about 2 medium bananas)

1 cup all-purpose flour

1 cup whole-wheat flour

1 teaspoon baking powder

½ teaspoon baking soda

2 teaspoons pumpkin pie spice

½ cup raisins

¼ cup chopped walnuts

Preheat the oven to 350°F. Spray a 5 × 9-inch loaf pan with nonstick cooking spray.

Mix the yogurt, brown sugar, egg substitute, lemon juice, and oil until smooth. Stir the bananas into the yogurt mixture.

In a separate bowl, combine the flours, baking powder, baking soda, and pumpkin pie spice. Fold the dry ingredients into the banana mixture, but do not overstir. Fold in the raisins and nuts, mixing gently.

Bake in the preheated oven for about 50 minutes or until golden brown and a toothpick inserted into the middle comes out clean. Remove the baked bread from the pan and let cool on a wire rack. When the bread is cool, cut into 10 slices.

Servings	Calories per serving	Fat (g)	Sodium (mg)
10 (¾-inch-thick slice each)	228	5	137

	Vegetables	Fruits/Juices	Dairy Foods	Grains
Food Group Serving(s):				1

	Meat, Poultry, and Fish	Nuts, Seeds, and Legumes	Added Fats/Oils	Sweets
Food Group Serving(s):				

Lemon Muffins

―――――――――――⋀―――――――――――

Dry Ingredients
1¾ cups all-purpose flour
¾ cup granulated sugar
1 teaspoon baking soda

Wet Ingredients
1 cup plain nonfat yogurt
3 tablespoons margarine

1 medium egg
1 tablespoon lemon juice
1 tablespoon grated lemon
   zest
¼ teaspoon lemon extract

Preheat the oven to 350°F. Spray a 12-cup muffin pan with nonstick cooking spray.

In separate bowls, combine the dry and wet ingredients. Mix the wet and dry ingredients together until just combined. Evenly divide the batter among the 12 muffin cups. Bake in the preheated oven for 12 to 15 minutes.

Servings	Calories per serving	Fat (g)	Sodium (mg)
12 (1 muffin each)	157	3.4	122

	Vegetables	Fruits/Juices	Dairy Foods	Grains
Food Group Serving(s):				1

	Meat, Poultry, and Fish	Nuts, Seeds, and Legumes	Added Fats/Oils	Sweets
Food Group Serving(s):				

Lighter Sweet Country Corn Bread

————————⌄————————

1 cup skim milk

2 tablespoons margarine, melted

2 egg whites

1¼ cups yellow cornmeal

1 cup all-purpose flour

½ cup granulated sugar

3 teaspoons low-sodium baking powder

Preheat the oven to 400°F. Grease the bottom and sides of an 8 × 8-inch pan with cooking spray.

In a large stainless steel mixing bowl, beat the milk, margarine, and egg whites together. Add the cornmeal, flour, sugar, and baking powder all at once and stir just until moistened (the batter will be lumpy). Pour the batter into the pan and bake for 20 to 25 minutes or until golden brown and a toothpick inserted in the center comes out dry.

Servings	Calories per serving	Fat (g)	Sodium (mg)
12 (2 x 2½-inch piece each)	144	2	45

	Vegetables	Fruits/Juices	Dairy Foods	Grains
Food Group Serving(s):				1

	Meat, Poultry, and Fish	Nuts, Seeds, and Legumes	Added Fats/Oils	Sweets
Food Group Serving(s):				

Quick Pumpkin Bread

―――――⌄―――――

2 cups reduced-fat pancake
   mix

¾ cup granulated sugar

½ teaspoon pumpkin pie spice

½ teaspoon ground cinnamon

1½ cups canned pumpkin

½ cup egg substitute or 4 egg
   whites

½ cup coarsely chopped
   Craisins

⅓ cup chopped walnuts

Preheat the oven to 350°F. Spray a 5 × 9-inch loaf pan with nonstick cooking spray.

In a large stainless steel mixing bowl, combine the pancake mix, sugar, pumpkin pie spice, and cinnamon. Set aside.

In another mixing bowl, combine the pumpkin and egg substitute. Add the dry ingredients, along with the Craisins and nuts, and stir just until combined. Pour the batter into the loaf pan.

Bake in the preheated oven for 50 minutes or until a wooden toothpick inserted into the center comes out clean.

Servings	Calories per serving	Fat (g)	Sodium (mg)
12 (¾-inch-thick slice each)	206	4	321

	Vegetables	Fruits/Juices	Dairy Foods	Grains
Food Group Serving(s):				1

	Meat, Poultry, and Fish	Nuts, Seeds, and Legumes	Added Fats/Oils	Sweets
Food Group Serving(s):				

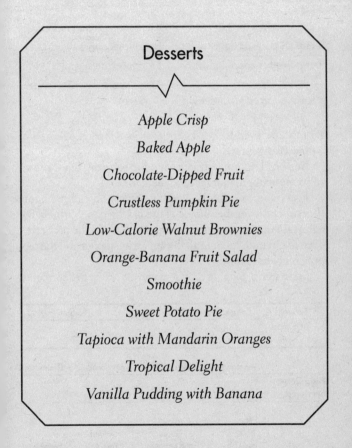

Desserts

Apple Crisp

Baked Apple

Chocolate-Dipped Fruit

Crustless Pumpkin Pie

Low-Calorie Walnut Brownies

Orange-Banana Fruit Salad

Smoothie

Sweet Potato Pie

Tapioca with Mandarin Oranges

Tropical Delight

Vanilla Pudding with Banana

Apple Crisp

―――――――∧―――――――

¼ cup instant oatmeal

¼ cup all-purpose flour

⅓ cup firmly packed light
  brown sugar

½ teaspoon ground cinnamon

¼ teaspoon ground nutmeg

1½ tablespoons margarine

4 Granny Smith apples

2 cups vanilla nonfat frozen
  yogurt

Preheat the oven to 375°F. Spray an 8 × 8-inch baking pan
with cooking spray.

In a bowl, thoroughly combine the oatmeal, flour, brown
sugar, cinnamon, nutmeg, and margarine.

Peel, core, and thinly slice the apples. Spread the apple
slices evenly over the surface of the baking pan. Sprinkle the
oatmeal-flour mixture over the apples. Bake in the preheated
oven for 30 minutes or until the apples are tender and the topping is golden brown.

Serve warm, topping each serving with ¼ cup frozen yogurt.

Servings	Calories per serving	Fat (g)	Sodium (mg)
8 (½ apple each)	108	2	53

	Vegetables	Fruits/Juices	Dairy Foods	Grains
Food Group Serving(s):		0.5		

	Meat, Poultry, and Fish	Nuts, Seeds, and Legumes	Added Fats/Oils	Sweets
Food Group Serving(s):				1

Baked Apple

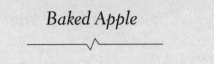

| 1 medium apple (Cortland) | ½ teaspoon ground cinnamon |
| ¼ teaspoon light brown sugar | 1 teaspoon chopped walnuts |

Core the apple and peel ⅓ of the way down from the top.

Place the apple in a baking dish and sprinkle the brown sugar, cinnamon, and walnuts over the top ⅓ and into the center. Microwave on high for 4 to 5 minutes or until the apple is tender when pierced with the tip of a thin-bladed knife.

Servings	Calories per serving	Fat (g)	Sodium (mg)
1	102	1	

	Vegetables	Fruits/Juices	Dairy Foods	Grains
Food Group Serving(s):		1		

	Meat, Poultry, and Fish	Nuts, Seeds, and Legumes	Added Fats/Oils	Sweets
Food Group Serving(s):				

Chocolate-Dipped Fruit

—————⋁—————

½ cup light chocolate syrup   1 cup canned pineapple
1 medium banana   chunks in juice, drained
12 medium strawberries

Place the chocolate syrup in a small dish for dipping.
    Peel and slice the banana. Arrange with the other fruit on
a plate. Serve with toothpicks or small forks.

Servings	Calories per serving	Fat (g)	Sodium (mg)
4 (¾ cup each)	111	1	49

	Vegetables	Fruits/Juices	Dairy Foods	Grains
Food Group Serving(s):		1.5		

	Meat, Poultry, and Fish	Nuts, Seeds, and Legumes	Added Fats/Oils	Sweets
Food Group Serving(s):				1

Crustless Pumpkin Pie

———⋀———

2 large eggs

1 (15-ounce) can solid-pack
pumpkin

¼ cup granulated sugar

2 teaspoons pumpkin pie
spice

¼ cup light molasses

1 teaspoon vanilla extract

1½ cups evaporated skim milk

6 tablespoons fat-free
whipped topping

Preheat the oven to 450°F. Spray a 10-inch pie plate with
nonstick cooking spray.

In a stainless steel mixing bowl, beat the eggs. Add the
pumpkin, sugar, pumpkin pie spice, molasses, and vanilla
and mix together. Gradually stir in the milk until thoroughly
incorporated.

Pour the mixture into the pie plate. Bake in the preheated
oven for 10 minutes. Lower the oven temperature to 350°F
and bake an additional 40 minutes or until a butter knife inserted in the center comes out clean. Top each serving with 1
tablespoon of light whipped topping.

Servings	Calories per serving	Fat (g)	Sodium (mg)
6 (⅙ of pie each)	169	2	100

	Vegetables	Fruits/Juices	Dairy Foods	Grains
Food Group Serving(s):	0.5		0.5	

	Meat, Poultry, and Fish	Nuts, Seeds, and Legumes	Added Fats/Oils	Sweets
Food Group Serving(s):				1

Low-Calorie Walnut Brownies

6 ounces semisweet chocolate ⅔ cup granulated sugar

½ cup hot water 1½ cups all-purpose flour

4 egg whites 1 teaspoon baking powder

1 teaspoon vanilla extract ½ cup chopped walnuts

Preheat the oven to 350°F. Spray an 8 × 8-inch cake pan with nonstick cooking spray.

In a large heatproof bowl set over simmering water, melt the chocolate with the hot water, stirring until smooth. Remove from the heat and let cool slightly. Whisk in the egg whites and mix in the vanilla. In a separate bowl, mix together the sugar, flour, and baking powder; stir into the chocolate batter until just combined. Stir in the walnuts. Pour the butter into the cake pan.

Bake for 20 to 30 minutes or until the edges pull away from the pan. Let cool on a rack, then serve.

Servings	Calories per serving	Fat (g)	Sodium (mg)
16 (2 x 2-inch piece each)	154	7	29

	Vegetables	Fruits/Juices	Dairy Foods	Grains
Food Group Serving(s):				

	Meat, Poultry, and Fish	Nuts, Seeds, and Legumes	Added Fats/Oils	Sweets
Food Group Serving(s):				1

Orange-Banana Fruit Salad

———— ⅄ ————

3 medium bananas

2 navel or other seedless oranges

⅛ teaspoon vanilla extract

Peel and slice the bananas into ½-inch-thick rounds. Peel and section the oranges. In a medium-size bowl, gently toss the fruit with the vanilla.

Servings	Calories per serving	Fat (g)	Sodium (mg)
4 (1½ cups each)	114	0.5	2

	Vegetables	Fruits/Juices	Dairy Foods	Grains
Food Group Serving(s):		1		

	Meat, Poultry, and Fish	Nuts, Seeds, and Legumes	Added Fats/Oils	Sweets
Food Group Serving(s):				

Smoothie

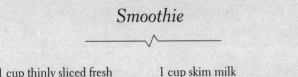

1 cup thinly sliced fresh strawberries (from about 10 strawberries)	1 cup skim milk
	1½ cups vanilla nonfat yogurt
1 very ripe medium banana, cut into small pieces	

Place the strawberries and banana in a blender with a small amount of milk and blend until smooth. Add the remaining milk and the yogurt and blend until well incorporated and creamy.

Servings	Calories per serving	Fat (g)	Sodium (mg)
3 (1¼ cups each)	141	1	108

	Vegetables	Fruits/Juices	Dairy Foods	Grains
Food Group Serving(s):		1	1	

	Meat, Poultry, and Fish	Nuts, Seeds, and Legumes	Added Fats/Oils	Sweets
Food Group Serving(s):				

Sweet Potato Pie

————————⋀————————

Crust

1¼ cups all-purpose flour

¼ teaspoon granulated sugar

⅓ cup skim milk

2 tablespoons canola oil

Filling

¼ cup granulated sugar

¼ cup firmly packed light
  brown sugar

¼ teaspoon salt

¼ teaspoon ground nutmeg

¾ cup egg substitute or 6 egg
  whites

¼ cup evaporated skim milk

1 teaspoon vanilla extract

3 cups cooked, mashed sweet
  potatoes (from about 2
  medium potatoes)

To make the crust, in a large stainless steel mixing bowl, combine the flour and sugar. Add the milk and oil and stir with a fork until well mixed. Turn the mixture out onto a floured work surface and knead it into a smooth ball. Roll out the dough to a thickness of ¼ inch and place in a 9-inch pie pan, patting to spread evenly.

Preheat the oven to 350°F.

To make the filling, in a large stainless steel mixing bowl, combine the sugars, salt, nutmeg, and egg substitute. Add the milk and vanilla and stir to incorporate. Add the sweet potatoes and mix well using an electric mixer.

Pour the mixture into the pie shell. Bake for 1 hour or until the crust is golden brown. Cool and cut into 16 small slices, making a rich, dense dish.

Servings	Calories per serving	Fat (g)	Sodium (mg)
16 (1/16 of pie each)	135	2	105

	Vegetables	Fruits/Juices	Dairy Foods	Grains
Food Group Serving(s):	0.5			

	Meat, Poultry, and Fish	Nuts, Seeds, and Legumes	Added Fats/Oils	Sweets
Food Group Serving(s):				1

Tapioca with Mandarin Oranges

———————— /\ ————————

3 tablespoons quick-cooking
    tapioca pudding mix

⅓ cup granulated sugar

2¾ cups skim milk

1 medium egg

1 teaspoon vanilla extract

1 cup canned mandarin
    oranges in light syrup,
    drained

Make the tapioca as directed on the box, using sugar, milk, egg, and vanilla. Let cool for 20 minutes.

Gently fold the mandarin oranges into the pudding. Divide the pudding among 8 custard bowls. Serve warm or refrigerate and serve chilled.

Servings	Calories per serving	Fat (g)	Sodium (mg)
8 (½ cups each)	104	1	49

	Vegetables	Fruits/Juices	Dairy Foods	Grains
Food Group Serving(s):				

	Meat, Poultry, and Fish	Nuts, Seeds, and Legumes	Added Fats/Oils	Sweets
Food Group Serving(s):				1

Tropical Delight

———————⌄———————

1 cup 1% low-fat cottage
  cheese
1 cup fat-free whipped
  topping
1 (3-ounce) box sugar-free
  orange-flavored gelatin
  mix

1 cup canned mandarin
  oranges in light syrup,
  drained
1 cup canned crushed
  pineapple, drained
¼ cup slivered almonds

Mix the cottage cheese, whipped topping, and dry gelatin mix. Stir in the oranges, pineapple, and almonds. Chill for at least 2 hours.

Servings	Calories per serving	Fat (g)	Sodium (mg)
8 (¾ cup each)	126	2	159

	Vegetables	Fruits/Juices	Dairy Foods	Grains
Food Group Serving(s):		0.5		

	Meat, Poultry, and Fish	Nuts, Seeds, and Legumes	Added Fats/Oils	Sweets
Food Group Serving(s):				

Vanilla Pudding with Banana

———————⌄———————

1 (3-ounce) box instant sugar-
   free, fat-free vanilla instant
   pudding and pie mix
2 cups skim milk

1 cup banana slices (from
   about 1 large banana)

Prepare the pudding mix according to directions on the package, using the milk. Cool for 10 minutes. Gently fold in the sliced banana, then pour into 4 dessert bowls.
   Refrigerate until chilled.

Servings	Calories per serving	Fat (g)	Sodium (mg)
4 (½ cup each)	108	1	354

	Vegetables	Fruits/Juices	Dairy Foods	Grains
Food Group Serving(s):			0.5	

	Meat, Poultry, and Fish	Nuts, Seeds, and Legumes	Added Fats/Oils	Sweets
Food Group Serving(s):				

11

---‾∨‾---

DASH Meal Plans

When you are just starting on the DASH Diet, it can be a little difficult to plan and keep track of your food groups. In this chapter you will find a total of 10 breakfast, 13 lunch, and 24 dinner plans. These meal plans are examples of how you can put a meal together that follows the DASH recommendations. You can mix and match any breakfast, lunch, and dinner to make up a whole day's menu. (Items with an asterisk are recipes in this book.)

Breakfast

Breakfast 1:

1 cup apple juice
3 tablespoons raisins
⅔ cup shredded wheat
1 slice whole-wheat toast
1 teaspoon unsalted margarine
1 teaspoon jelly
1 cup skim milk

Calories per serving	Fat (g)	Sodium (mg)
533	6	294

	Vegetables	Fruits/Juices	Dairy Foods	Grains
Food Group Serving(s):		2	1	2

	Meat, Poultry, and Fish	Nuts, Seeds, and Legumes	Added Fats/Oils	Sweets
Food Group Serving(s):			1	1

Breakfast 2:

½ cup stewed prunes
1 cup cooked oatmeal
1 cup skim milk
½ cup fresh strawberries
1 slice whole-wheat bread
1 teaspoon unsalted margarine

Calories per serving	Fat (g)	Sodium (mg)
491	8	281

	Vegetables	Fruits/Juices	Dairy Foods	Grains
Food Group Serving(s):		2	1	2

	Meat, Poultry, and Fish	Nuts, Seeds, and Legumes	Added Fats/Oils	Sweets
Food Group Serving(s):			1	

Breakfast 3:

1 cup orange juice
½ cup cantaloupe cubes
½ whole-wheat bagel
1 tablespoon fat-free cream cheese
2 teaspoons jelly
1 cup skim milk

Calories per serving	Fat (g)	Sodium (mg)
419	2	490

	Vegetables	Fruits/Juices	Dairy Foods	Grains
Food Group Serving(s):		2	1	1

	Meat, Poultry, and Fish	Nuts, Seeds, and Legumes	Added Fats/Oils	Sweets
Food Group Serving(s):				1

Breakfast 4:

1 cup orange juice
¼ cup banana slices
¼ cup strawberries
1 toasted English muffin
1 tablespoon almond butter
8 ounces plain nonfat yogurt

Calories per serving	Fat (g)	Sodium (mg)
513	11	397

	Vegetables	Fruits/Juices	Dairy Foods	Grains
Food Group Serving(s):		2	1	2

	Meat, Poultry, and Fish	Nuts, Seeds, and Legumes	Added Fats/Oils	Sweets
Food Group Serving(s):		0.5		

Breakfast 5:

1 cup orange juice
1 medium peach
2 oatmeal-raisin granola bars
1 slice whole-wheat toast
1 teaspoon unsalted margarine
1 cup skim milk

Calories per serving	Fat (g)	Sodium (mg)
562	10	416

	Vegetables	Fruits/Juices	Dairy Foods	Grains
Food Group Serving(s):		2	1	3

	Meat, Poultry, and Fish	Nuts, Seeds, and Legumes	Added Fats/Oils	Sweets
Food Group Serving(s):			1	

Breakfast 6:

1 cup orange juice
½ cup cantaloupe cubes
1 cinnamon-raisin bagel
1 tablespoon fat-free cream cheese
1 tablespoon orange marmalade
1 cup skim milk

Calories per serving	Fat (g)	Sodium (mg)	
486	2	456	

	Vegetables	Fruits/Juices	Dairy Foods	Grains
Food Group Serving(s):		2	1	2

	Meat, Poultry, and Fish	Nuts, Seeds, and Legumes	Added Fats/Oils	Sweets
Food Group Serving(s):				1

Breakfast 7:

1 cup orange juice
½ grapefruit
2 servings Blueberry Pancakes*
1 tablespoon maple syrup
1 cup skim milk

Calories per serving	Fat (g)	Sodium (mg)	
550	3	427	

	Vegetables	Fruits/Juices	Dairy Foods	Grains
Food Group Serving(s):		2	1	2

	Meat, Poultry, and Fish	Nuts, Seeds, and Legumes	Added Fats/Oils	Sweets
Food Group Serving(s):				1

Breakfast 8:

1 cup orange juice
1 banana
1 poached egg
1 Lemon Muffin*
1 cup skim milk

Calories per serving	Fat (g)	Sodium (mg)
537	10	392

	Vegetables	Fruits/Juices	Dairy Foods	Grains
Food Group Serving(s):		2	1	1

	Meat, Poultry, and Fish	Nuts, Seeds, and Legumes	Added Fats/Oils	Sweets
Food Group Serving(s):	1			

Breakfast 9:

1 cup orange juice
½ cup raspberries
¾ cup Frosted Mini Wheats
1 slice whole-wheat toast
1 teaspoon unsalted margarine
1 cup skim milk

Calories per serving	Fat (g)	Sodium (mg)
470	7	278

	Vegetables	Fruits/Juices	Dairy Foods	Grains
Food Group Serving(s):		2	1	2

	Meat, Poultry, and Fish	Nuts, Seeds, and Legumes	Added Fats/Oils	Sweets
Food Group Serving(s):			1	

Breakfast 10:

1 cup orange juice
1 slice whole-wheat toast
1 teaspoon unsalted margarine
1 serving Apple Cobbler*
1 cup skim milk

Calories per serving	Fat (g)	Sodium (mg)
470	7	284

	Vegetables	Fruits/Juices	Dairy Foods	Grains
Food Group Serving(s):		2	1	2

	Meat, Poultry, and Fish	Nuts, Seeds, and Legumes	Added Fats/Oils	Sweets
Food Group Serving(s):			1	

Lunch

Lunch 1:

1 serving Broccoli and Walnut Salad*
4 slices tomato
6 pieces romaine lettuce
1 whole-wheat pita pocket
¾ cup plain nonfat yogurt
¾ cup pineapple tidbits

Calories per serving	Fat (g)	Sodium (mg)
647	18	503

	Vegetables	Fruits/Juices	Dairy Foods	Grains
Food Group Serving(s):	4	2	1	2

	Meat, Poultry, and Fish	Nuts, Seeds, and Legumes	Added Fats/Oils	Sweets
Food Group Serving(s):				

Lunch 2:

1 serving Hawaiian Chicken Sandwich*
1 serving Tomato and Red Onion Salad*
1 serving Smoothie*

Calories per serving	Fat (g)	Sodium (mg)
600	11	523

	Vegetables	Fruits/Juices	Dairy Foods	Grains
Food Group Serving(s):	3	1	1	3

	Meat, Poultry, and Fish	Nuts, Seeds, and Legumes	Added Fats/Oils	Sweets
Food Group Serving(s):	1			

Lunch 3:

Roast Beef Sandwich:
    2 ounces roast beef, trimmed
    1 teaspoon low-sodium barbecue sauce
    2 slices mixed-grain bread

Salad:
    ½ cup chopped romaine lettuce
    ½ cup chopped tomato
    ¼ cup chopped green bell pepper
    1 tablespoon low-sodium diet Italian salad dressing
    1 baked potato, cut into bite-size pieces and placed on top
      of salad

1 medium apple
1 cup skim milk

Calories per serving	Fat (g)	Sodium (mg)
593	9	581

	Vegetables	Fruits/Juices	Dairy Foods	Grains
Food Group Serving(s):	3	1	1	2

	Meat, Poultry, and Fish	Nuts, Seeds, and Legumes	Added Fats/Oils	Sweets
Food Group Serving(s):	1			

Lunch 4:

Chicken Sandwich:
    2 ounces cooked chicken breast
    2 slices whole-wheat bread
    1½ ounces low-sodium cheddar cheese
    ¼ cup shredded iceberg lettuce
    2 (¼-inch) slices tomato

10 baby carrots
¾ cup applesauce
1 medium banana

Calories per serving	Fat (g)	Sodium (mg)
777	27	394

	Vegetables	Fruits/Juices	Dairy Foods	Grains
Food Group Serving(s):	2	2	1	2

	Meat, Poultry, and Fish	Nuts, Seeds, and Legumes	Added Fats/Oils	Sweets
Food Group Serving(s):	1			

Lunch 5:

Tuna Fish Sandwich:
  2 ounces water-packed unsalted tuna
  2 slices whole-wheat bread
  2 teaspoons low-sodium light mayonnaise
  2 ounces low-sodium, low-fat cheese
  3 pieces romaine lettuce
  2 (¼-inch) tomato slices

½ cup steamed chopped broccoli
1 medium peach

Calories per serving	Fat (g)	Sodium (mg)
465	11	404

	Vegetables	Fruits/Juices	Dairy Foods	Grains
Food Group Serving(s):	2	1	1	2

	Meat, Poultry, and Fish	Nuts, Seeds, and Legumes	Added Fats/Oils	Sweets
Food Group Serving(s):	1		1	

Lunch 6:

Chicken Sandwich:
   2 ounces roasted chicken breast
   2 slices whole-wheat bread
   2 tablespoons low-sodium light mayonnaise
   3 pieces romaine lettuce
   2 (¼-inch) slices tomato

10 baby carrots
1 medium orange
1 cup skim milk
1 Jell-O gelatin snack

Calories per serving	Fat (g)	Sodium (mg)
577	12	628

	Vegetables	Fruits/Juices	Dairy Foods	Grains
Food Group Serving(s):	3.5	1	1	2

	Meat, Poultry, and Fish	Nuts, Seeds, and Legumes	Added Fats/Oils	Sweets
Food Group Serving(s):	1		2	1

Lunch 7:

Chicken Salad:
   ¼ cup chopped cooked chicken breast
   2 teaspoons low-sodium light mayonnaise
   ¼ cup shredded lettuce
   2 (¼-inch) slices tomato
   ⅛ cup sliced red onion
   ¼ cup alfalfa sprouts
   ½ whole-wheat pita pocket

1 serving Sweet-Potato Chips*
1 medium banana
1 cup skim milk

Calories per serving	Fat (g)	Sodium (mg)
516	8	599

	Vegetables	Fruits/Juices	Dairy Foods	Grains
Food Group Serving(s):	2	1	1	1

	Meat, Poultry, and Fish	Nuts, Seeds, and Legumes	Added Fats/Oils	Sweets
Food Group Serving(s):	1		1	

Lunch 8:

1 serving Couscous with Broccoli*
1 serving Quick Pumpkin Bread*
1 cup skim milk
1 medium banana

Calories per serving	Fat (g)	Sodium (mg)
691	8	472

	Vegetables	Fruits/Juices	Dairy Foods	Grains
Food Group Serving(s):	1	1	1	1.5

	Meat, Poultry, and Fish	Nuts, Seeds, and Legumes	Added Fats/Oils	Sweets
Food Group Serving(s):				

Lunch 9:

1 cup orange juice
1 serving Wild Rice Pilaf*
2 tablespoons low-sodium cheddar cheese
1 cup cooked mixed vegetables
½ cup frozen yogurt

Calories per serving	Fat (g)	Sodium (mg)
599	14	249

	Vegetables	Fruits/Juices	Dairy Foods	Grains
Food Group Serving(s):	2	1	1	1

	Meat, Poultry, and Fish	Nuts, Seeds, and Legumes	Added Fats/Oils	Sweets
Food Group Serving(s):				

Lunch 10:

1 cup orange juice
1 serving Swiss Cheese Sandwich*
½ cup watermelon balls

Calories per serving	Fat (g)	Sodium (mg)
485	15	390

	Vegetables	Fruits/Juices	Dairy Foods	Grains
Food Group Serving(s):	3.5	2	0.5	2

	Meat, Poultry, and Fish	Nuts, Seeds, and Legumes	Added Fats/Oils	Sweets
Food Group Serving(s):		1		

Lunch 11:

1 serving Tossed Salad I or II*
1 serving Tortellini and Bean Soup*
1 whole-wheat roll
1 serving Chocolate-Dipped Fruit*
1 cup skim milk

Calories per serving	Fat (g)	Sodium (mg)
556	8	515

	Vegetables	Fruits/Juices	Dairy Foods	Grains
Food Group Serving(s):	3.5	1.5	1.5	1.5

	Meat, Poultry, and Fish	Nuts, Seeds, and Legumes	Added Fats/Oils	Sweets
Food Group Serving(s):		1		1

Lunch 12:

1 serving Turkey Burger*
1 serving Coleslaw with Dates*
1 medium apple
1 cup skim milk

Calories per serving	Fat (g)	Sodium (mg)
568	16	676

	Vegetables	Fruits/Juices	Dairy Foods	Grains
Food Group Serving(s):	3	1.5	1	2

	Meat, Poultry, and Fish	Nuts, Seeds, and Legumes	Added Fats/Oils	Sweets
Food Group Serving(s):	0.5			

Lunch 13:

1 cup apple juice
1 serving Tomato-Orange Soup*
1 cup steamed green beans
2 whole-wheat rolls
1 teaspoon unsalted margarine
2 medium plums
½ cup skim milk

Calories per serving	Fat (g)	Sodium (mg)
536	9	497

	Vegetables	Fruits/Juices	Dairy Foods	Grains
Food Group Serving(s):	3	2	0.5	2

	Meat, Poultry, and Fish	Nuts, Seeds, and Legumes	Added Fats/Oils	Sweets
Food Group Serving(s):			1	

Dinner

Dinner 1:

1 serving Dave's Cajun Catfish*
½ serving New Orleans Red Beans and Rice*
½ cup steamed or boiled okra
2 servings Lighter Sweet Country Corn Bread*
1 serving Tossed Salad I*
1 teaspoon olive oil
1 tablespoon balsamic vinegar
½ fresh papaya
1 cup skim milk

Calories per serving	Fat (g)	Sodium (mg)
748	23	746

	Vegetables	Fruits/Juices	Dairy Foods	Grains
Food Group Serving(s):	3.5	1	1	2.5

	Meat, Poultry, and Fish	Nuts, Seeds, and Legumes	Added Fats/Oils	Sweets
Food Group Serving(s):	1	0.5	1	

Dinner 2:

1 serving Blackened Beef with Greens and Red Potatoes*
2 slices whole-wheat bread
1 cup plain nonfat yogurt
½ cup fruit cocktail

Calories per serving	Fat (g)	Sodium (mg)
866	13	618

	Vegetables	Fruits/Juices	Dairy Foods	Grains
Food Group Serving(s):	4	1	1	2

	Meat, Poultry, and Fish	Nuts, Seeds, and Legumes	Added Fats/Oils	Sweets
Food Group Serving(s):	1			

Dinner 3:

1 serving Grilled Tuna*
1 serving Wild Rice Pilaf*
1 serving Sautéed Collard Greens*
10 baby carrots
1 tablespoon fat-free ranch salad dressing
2 whole-wheat rolls
2 teaspoons unsalted margarine
1 serving Baked Apple*
1 cup skim milk

Calories per serving	Fat (g)	Sodium (mg)
882	23	775

	Vegetables	Fruits/Juices	Dairy Foods	Grains
Food Group Serving(s):	4	1	1	3

	Meat, Poultry, and Fish	Nuts, Seeds, and Legumes	Added Fats/Oils	Sweets
Food Group Serving(s):	1		2	

Dinner 4:

1½ cups Gingered Butternut Squash Soup*
1½ cups Tossed Salad I or II*
2 cherry tomatoes
2 tablespoons shredded low-sodium cheddar cheese
2 tablespoons low-sodium French salad dressing
2 whole-wheat rolls
2 teaspoons unsalted margarine
1 cup orange juice

Calories per serving	Fat (g)	Sodium (mg)
805	34	910

	Vegetables	Fruits/Juices	Dairy Foods	Grains
Food Group Serving(s):	3.5	1	1	2

	Meat, Poultry, and Fish	Nuts, Seeds, and Legumes	Added Fats/Oils	Sweets
Food Group Serving(s):		1.5	3	

Dinner 5:

1 serving Baked Catfish*
1 serving Hot Red Potato and Spinach Salad*
½ cup steamed chopped broccoli
2 whole-wheat rolls
2 teaspoons unsalted margarine
1 cup vanilla low-fat yogurt
1 medium peach

Calories per serving	Fat (g)	Sodium (mg)
821	21	904

	Vegetables	Fruits/Juices	Dairy Foods	Grains
Food Group Serving(s):	3	1	1	2

	Meat, Poultry, and Fish	Nuts, Seeds, and Legumes	Added Fats/Oils	Sweets
Food Group Serving(s):	1	0.5	2	

Dinner 6:

1 serving Fettuccine with Chicken and Vegetables*
1 serving Soybean Salad*
1 cup steamed green beans
2 slices Italian bread
1 teaspoon unsalted margarine
¼ cup cubed cantaloupe
¼ cup cubed papaya
¼ cup banana slices
½ cup low-fat frozen yogurt

Calories per serving	Fat (g)	Sodium (mg)
863	19	663

	Vegetables	Fruits/Juices	Dairy Foods	Grains
Food Group Serving(s):	3.5	1.5	1	3

	Meat, Poultry, and Fish	Nuts, Seeds, and Legumes	Added Fats/Oils	Sweets
Food Group Serving(s):	0.5	1.5	1	

Dinner 7:

1 serving Grilled Tuna*
1 serving Bulgur Wheat with Tomatoes*
1 serving Sautéed Collard Greens*
1 serving Quick Pumpkin Bread*
½ cup plain low-fat yogurt
1 cup apple juice

Calories per serving	Fat (g)	Sodium (mg)
822	13	538

	Vegetables	Fruits/Juices	Dairy Foods	Grains
Food Group Serving(s):	4.5	1	0.5	2

	Meat, Poultry, and Fish	Nuts, Seeds, and Legumes	Added Fats/Oils	Sweets
Food Group Serving(s):	1			

Dinner 8:

1 serving Snapper with Greens*
1 medium baked potato
2 tablespoons salsa
2 tablespoons plain low-fat yogurt
½ serving Fresh Fruit Salad*
½ cup citrus fruit sorbet
2 whole-wheat rolls

Calories per serving	Fat (g)	Sodium (mg)
683	8	741

	Vegetables	Fruits/Juices	Dairy Foods	Grains
Food Group Serving(s):	4	1	0.5	2

	Meat, Poultry, and Fish	Nuts, Seeds, and Legumes	Added Fats/Oils	Sweets
Food Group Serving(s):	1			

Dinner 9:

1 serving Sweet-and-Sour Pork with Vegetables*
1 cup cooked brown rice
1 serving Cherry Tomato and Scallion Salad*
2 teaspoons fresh lemon juice
1 serving Vanilla Pudding with Banana*
½ cup skim milk

Calories per serving	Fat (g)	Sodium (mg)
849	25	772

	Vegetables	Fruits/Juices	Dairy Foods	Grains
Food Group Serving(s):	3	0.5	1	2

	Meat, Poultry, and Fish	Nuts, Seeds, and Legumes	Added Fats/Oils	Sweets
Food Group Serving(s):	0.5	0.5		

Dinner 10:

1 serving Chicken Fruity Stir-fry*
½ cup cooked brown rice
½ cup steamed green peas

1 serving Stuffed Acorn Squash*
¾ cup plain nonfat yogurt
½ medium banana

Calories per serving	Fat (g)	Sodium (mg)
852	13	308

	Vegetables	Fruits/Juices	Dairy Foods	Grains
Food Group Serving(s):	3	2	1	1

	Meat, Poultry, and Fish	Nuts, Seeds, and Legumes	Added Fats/Oils	Sweets
Food Group Serving(s):	0.5			

Dinner 11:

1 cup orange juice
1 serving Northeast Gumbo*
1 cup cooked brown rice
1 serving Tossed Salad I or II*
1 teaspoon olive oil
1 tablespoon balsamic vinegar
3 tablespoons shredded cheddar cheese
1 serving Apple Crisp*

Calories per serving	Fat (g)	Sodium (mg)
885	26	449

	Vegetables	Fruits/Juices	Dairy Foods	Grains
Food Group Serving(s):	3.5	1.5	0.5	2

	Meat, Poultry, and Fish	Nuts, Seeds, and Legumes	Added Fats/Oils	Sweets
Food Group Serving(s):	1	1.5	1	1

Dinner 12:

1 serving Vermont Roast with Brown Mustard*
1 serving Baked Brown Bread*
1 serving Tossed Salad I*
1 teaspoon olive oil
1 tablespoon balsamic vinegar
1 cup low-fat frozen yogurt
½ cup strawberries

Calories per serving	Fat (g)	Sodium (mg)
926	20	567

	Vegetables	Fruits/Juices	Dairy Foods	Grains
Food Group Serving(s):	4.5	1	2	1

	Meat, Poultry, and Fish	Nuts, Seeds, and Legumes	Added Fats/Oils	Sweets
Food Group Serving(s):	1		1	

Dinner 13:

1 serving Baked Macaroni and Cheese*
1 serving Tossed Salad I*
1 tablespoon low-sodium French salad dressing
1 serving Green Beans with Almonds*
2 whole-wheat rolls
1 teaspoon unsalted margarine

1 serving Orange-Banana Fruit Salad*
½ cup orange juice

Calories per serving	Fat (g)	Sodium (mg)
889	31	749

	Vegetables	Fruits/Juices	Dairy Foods	Grains
Food Group Serving(s):	3	1.5	1	3

	Meat, Poultry, and Fish	Nuts, Seeds, and Legumes	Added Fats/Oils	Sweets
Food Group Serving(s):			1	

Dinner 14:

Vegetarian Spaghetti:
     ⅔ cup Vegetarian Spaghetti Sauce*
     1 cup cooked spaghetti
     1 cup cooked turnip greens
     3 tablespoons low-sodium Parmesan cheese

Salad:
     1 cup chopped raw spinach
     2 cherry tomatoes
     1 slice red onion
     1 tablespoon fat-free Italian salad dressing

1 whole-wheat roll
1 teaspoon unsalted margarine
1 serving Orange-Banana Fruit Salad*

Calories per serving	Fat (g)	Sodium (mg)
653	17	594

	Vegetables	Fruits/Juices	Dairy Foods	Grains
Food Group Serving(s):	4	1	1	3

	Meat, Poultry, and Fish	Nuts, Seeds, and Legumes	Added Fats/Oils	Sweets
Food Group Serving(s):			1	

Dinner 15:

4 ounces baked or broiled salmon fillet
1 cup cooked brown rice
1 serving Broccoli Rabe*
1 serving Three-Bean Salad*
1 serving Lighter Sweet Country Corn Bread*
1 serving Smoothie*

Calories per serving	Fat (g)	Sodium (mg)
863	20	579

	Vegetables	Fruits/Juices	Dairy Foods	Grains
Food Group Serving(s):	3	1	1	3

	Meat, Poultry, and Fish	Nuts, Seeds, and Legumes	Added Fats/Oils	Sweets
Food Group Serving(s):	1	1.5		

Dinner 16:

1 serving Chicken with Rice*
1 cup steamed green peas
2 servings Lighter Sweet Country Corn Bread*

2 teaspoons unsalted margarine
1 cup cantaloupe chunks
1 cup skim milk

Calories per serving	Fat (g)	Sodium (mg)
878	26	431

	Vegetables	Fruits/Juices	Dairy Foods	Grains
Food Group Serving(s):	3	2	1	3.5

	Meat, Poultry, and Fish	Nuts, Seeds, and Legumes	Added Fats/Oils	Sweets
Food Group Serving(s):	1		2	

Dinner 17:

1 serving Chicken and Broccoli Bake*
1 serving Cherry Tomato and Scallion Salad*
1 cup cooked brown rice
1 teaspoon unsalted margarine
1 serving Crustless Pumpkin Pie*
1 cup orange juice

Calories per serving	Fat (g)	Sodium (mg)
878	20	470

	Vegetables	Fruits/Juices	Dairy Foods	Grains
Food Group Serving(s):	4.5	1	1.5	2

	Meat, Poultry, and Fish	Nuts, Seeds, and Legumes	Added Fats/Oils	Sweets
Food Group Serving(s):	0.5		1	1

Dinner 18:

1 serving Spicy Cod*
1 serving Scallion Rice*
½ cup steamed sliced carrots
1 serving Kale with Sesame Seeds*
1 dinner roll
½ cup cantaloupe chunks
1 cup skim milk

Calories per serving	Fat (g)	Sodium (mg)
982	26	539

	Vegetables	Fruits/Juices	Dairy Foods	Grains
Food Group Serving(s):	2.5	1	1	3

	Meat, Poultry, and Fish	Nuts, Seeds, and Legumes	Added Fats/Oils	Sweets
Food Group Serving(s):	1			

Dinner 19:

3 ounces trimmed beef chuck roast
½ medium baked potato
1 tablespoon nonfat sour cream
¾ cup steamed green beans
1 multigrain sandwich roll
1 medium peach
1 cup plain low-fat yogurt
2 tablespoons unsalted roasted peanuts

Calories per serving	Fat (g)	Sodium (mg)
896	25	584

	Vegetables	Fruits/Juices	Dairy Foods	Grains
Food Group **Serving(s):**	2.5	1	1	2

	Meat, Poultry, and Fish	Nuts, Seeds, and Legumes	Added Fats/Oils	Sweets
Food Group **Serving(s):**	1	0.5		

Dinner 20:

1 serving Vegetarian Lasagna*
½ cup steamed spinach
½ cup steamed sliced carrots
2 dinner rolls
1 teaspoon unsalted margarine
1 serving Low-Calorie Walnut Brownies*
1 cup orange juice

Calories per serving	Fat (g)	Sodium (mg)
736	21	707

	Vegetables	Fruits/Juices	Dairy Foods	Grains
Food Group **Serving(s):**	4	1	1	3

	Meat, Poultry, and Fish	Nuts, Seeds, and Legumes	Added Fats/Oils	Sweets
Food Group **Serving(s):**			1	1

Dinner 21:

1 serving BBQ Pork Chops*
1 cup cooked brown rice
1 serving Molasses-Braised Collards*

1 serving Spicy Carrot Salad*
1 serving Tropical Delight*
½ cup skim milk

Calories per serving	Fat (g)	Sodium (mg)	
871	22	544	

	Vegetables	Fruits/Juices	Dairy Foods	Grains
Food Group Serving(s):	4	0.5	1	2

	Meat, Poultry, and Fish	Nuts, Seeds, and Legumes	Added Fats/Oils	Sweets
Food Group Serving(s):	1			

Dinner 22:

1 serving Limas and Spinach*
1 serving Couscous with Broccoli*
2 whole-wheat rolls
1 teaspoon unsalted margarine
1 cup plain low-fat yogurt
½ cup banana slices

Calories per serving	Fat (g)	Sodium (mg)	
884	16	561	

	Vegetables	Fruits/Juices	Dairy Foods	Grains
Food Group Serving(s):	2.5	1	1	2.5

	Meat, Poultry, and Fish	Nuts, Seeds, and Legumes	Added Fats/Oils	Sweets
Food Group Serving(s):			1	

Dinner 23:

4 ounces cooked large shrimp
1 serving Mango and Black Bean Salad*
1 cup cooked zucchini slices
2 (6-inch) corn tortillas
1 cup plain low-fat yogurt
½ cup raspberries
2 tablespoons unsalted almonds

Calories per serving	Fat (g)	Sodium (mg)
809	22	516

	Vegetables	Fruits/Juices	Dairy Foods	Grains
Food Group Serving(s):	3	1	1	2

	Meat, Poultry, and Fish	Nuts, Seeds, and Legumes	Added Fats/Oils	Sweets
Food Group Serving(s):	1	1.5		

Dinner 24:

Chicken Salad:

   3 ounces roasted chicken breast, without skin, cubed
   2 cups chopped romaine lettuce
   ½ cup cherry tomatoes
   4 tablespoons low-fat shredded cheddar cheese
   2 slices large red onion
   1 tablespoon unsalted sunflower seeds
   1 tablespoon balsamic vinegar
   2 teaspoons olive oil

2 whole-wheat rolls
1 teaspoon unsalted margarine
1 serving Sweet Potato Pie*
1 cup orange juice

Calories per serving	Fat (g)	Sodium (mg)	
817	27	636	

	Vegetables	Fruits/Juices	Dairy Foods	Grains
Food Group Serving(s):	3.5	1	1	2

	Meat, Poultry, and Fish	Nuts, Seeds, and Legumes	Added Fats/Oils	Sweets
Food Group Serving(s):	1	0.5	1	1

Appendix A

―――――――――/\―――――――――

The Science Behind DASH

To create a diet that would lower blood pressure, we knew we needed to study people who have healthy blood pressure and incorporate into our diet the characteristics of their eating patterns. For this we turned to two main sources.

Non-Westernized peoples: In stark contrast to the United States, where one in four adults has hypertension and over half of people who reach the age of 60 develop high blood pressure, many non-Westernized populations have low rates of hypertension, and their people do not experience an increase in hypertension as they age.

Among the characteristics of these societies is a diet based on foods obtained primarily from subsistence agriculture, fishing, and hunting. Most often the diet is high in fruits, vegetables, and fish. How we know that diet plays an important role in hypertension is that when populations with low rates of high blood pressure become urbanized and start eating more processed food and less fresh food, their rates of hypertension climb. This has been observed in South African Bantu natives, Bedouins in the Arabian desert, Aborigines in Australia, and Greenlanders.

Vegetarians in Westernized/urbanized societies: In modern America, where high blood pressure is prevalent, there is a group of people defined by what they eat who tend to have lower rates of high blood pressure: vegetarians. Although vegetarianism can take various forms, vegetarians can generally be said to eat a diet high in whole grains, beans, vegetables, and sometimes fish, dairy foods, eggs, and fruit.

In one study the rates of hypertension in Benedictine monks were compared to those of Trappist monks. The results showed that 30 percent of the Benedictine order had hypertension, while only 12 percent of the Trappists had the condition. Why is this significant? Because Benedictine monks eat meat, and Trappist monks are vegetarian.

Both non-Westernized peoples and vegetarians in Westernized/urbanized societies tend to have healthy blood pressure, and it seems certain that diet plays a central role in keeping their blood pressure that way. What the diets of both groups have in common is that they are high in plant foods (grains, nuts, seeds, vegetables, and sometimes fruit) and low in animal products (although sometimes high in fish consumption). Nutrient-wise, the diets are rich in the minerals potassium, magnesium, and calcium; high in fiber; and low in saturated fats.

Our goal was to create a diet with these same characteristics that would be acceptable to the average American and would not require that people become vegetarians. The DASH diet is such a diet. It does not prohibit any particular foods nor insist that you focus on any one food group. Yet the DASH diet has *two-and-a-half times* the amounts of potassium, magnesium, and calcium as the average American diet; *three times* as much dietary fiber; and less saturated fat, total fat, and cholesterol.

The Role of Key Nutrients in Keeping Blood Pressure Healthy

We don't really know how the DASH diet lowers blood pressure; we only know that it does. But we designed the diet to provide liberal amounts of several key nutrients that past medical studies have shown help lower blood pressure. In this section we'll review some of that evidence for you, but remember, you don't have to keep track of any complicated mineral amounts to follow the DASH diet. The DASH diet is about whole foods, things you recognize in the grocery store, like orange juice, tomatoes, milk, carrots, and a lot of other common, delicious, and healthful foods. This section is for your reading pleasure. You don't have to memorize it to be successful on the DASH diet.

Your body needs minerals to build, maintain, and repair itself. Although you need to consume only small quantities of even the most important minerals, your body won't work correctly without adequate amounts of these key substances.

Research has shown that insufficient intake of dietary potassium and perhaps magnesium and calcium may cause you to develop high blood pressure. In people who have hypertension, eating a diet rich in these key minerals is an important step toward lowering their blood pressure to healthier levels.

Potassium

Populations who eat a diet high in potassium generally have a low rate of hypertension, and when potassium-rich foods are given to study participants, blood pressure usually drops. In a typical study, an increase in potassium equal to three servings of fruits and vegetables caused a decrease of 2 to 3 mm Hg in blood pressure. Potassium supplements in pill form have been more successful than other nutrient supplements in lowering blood pressure in study participants, especially African-Americans and people who eat a very salty diet. Potassium isn't the only reason DASH lowers blood pressure, but it certainly contributes to the DASH effect.

It appears that potassium not only has a direct role in lowering blood pressure but may also prevent the consequences of hypertension, such as stroke and heart attack. In 2000 the Food and Drug Administration (FDA) recommended a diet high in potassium as a way to reduce the risk of high blood pressure and stroke.

Potassium enables your muscles to work properly. And not just the big muscles—it is also crucial for the proper function of the tiny muscle cells in your blood vessel walls. Potassium relaxes these muscle cells and opens up the blood vessels. In scientific language, it is a vasodilator (*vaso* refers to the blood vessels, or arteries and veins; *dilator* means "to make wider or expand"). The job potassium does is similar to that of important blood pressure medications also known as vasodilators.

Another reason potassium is important for blood pressure is that it helps the body get rid of sodium in the urine (excess sodium in your body raises blood pressure). It also facilitates the job done by the minerals calcium and magnesium in keeping blood pressure healthy.

Despite the positive effect potassium has on blood pressure and other areas of our health, most Americans don't get enough of this mineral in their diet. Nutritionists generally recommend you get at least 3,500 milligrams of potassium in your diet every day, and yet the average American has a daily intake of only about 1,800 milligrams.

By eating the DASH diet, you will consume 4,500 milligrams of potassium every day in a diet of whole foods. Why 4,500 milligrams? We chose this amount by looking at how much potassium is in the diet of populations with low rates of hypertension. Foods rich in potassium include almost all fruits, fruit juices, and vegetables, as well as dairy products. Also high in potassium are blackstrap molasses, brown rice, and whole grains.

Not all fruits and vegetables are equally rich in potassium. The DASH diet favors those that tend to have a higher potassium content. The list below ranks the best food sources of potassium, with the amount of potassium in parentheses.

Potassium All-Stars

- potato, baked with skin, 7 oz. (703 mg)
- yogurt, low-fat vanilla, 8 oz. (498 mg)
- banana (467 mg)
- orange juice, 1 cup (450 mg)
- milk, 1 cup (406 mg)
- grapefruit juice, canned, 1 cup (405 mg)
- acorn squash, boiled, mashed, ½ cup (321 mg)
- spinach, raw, 1 cup (312 mg)
- strawberries, 1 cup (247 mg)
- broccoli, chopped, boiled, ½ cup (228 mg)
- chickpeas, canned, ½ cup (207 mg)
- watermelon, balls, 1 cup (186 mg)

Calcium

Experts have long believed that there is a relationship between calcium intake and blood pressure. Although positive relationships between calcium and healthy blood pressure have been recorded in studies of populations that get a lot of calcium in their diets, trying to replicate these beneficial effects in controlled settings has been difficult, and the results have been inconsistent. Giving study participants calcium supplements in pill form has not been successful. When calcium supplementation has worked, the improvements in blood pressure health have been only modest. It is clear that calcium by itself is not sufficient to lower blood pressure, but as part of the DASH diet, it may contribute to DASH's blood-pressure-lowering effect.

Scientists theorize that calcium keeps blood pressure down because it helps relax the arteries and reduces the blood volume in the veins. In addition, calcium—like potassium—encourages the body to get rid of sodium in the urine.

The evidence suggests there *is* a relationship between calcium and blood pressure: sufficient amounts of calcium in your diet contribute to healthy blood pressure, and not enough dietary calcium can cause hypertension. Still, most Americans don't get nearly enough calcium in their diet. The average American consumes only about 450 milligrams of calcium per day—less than half of what is recommended. This deficiency may explain why hypertension levels in the United States are so high. By eating the DASH diet, you will consume 1,200 milligrams of calcium in your diet every day in whole foods. Why 1,200 milligrams? We chose this amount by looking at how much calcium is in the diet of populations with low rates of hypertension. Luckily, this is also the amount of calcium recommended to keep bones healthy and prevent osteoporosis.

Your most important source of calcium is dairy products. Milk, yogurt, and cheese are rich sources of calcium, and they are readily available and easy to incorporate into your diet. In addition, there's evidence that other nutrients in dairy products, such as phosphorus and protein, may combine with calcium to make dairy products especially effective at lowering blood pressure. Foods other than dairy products also contain calcium: sardines with bones, clams, bok choy, collard greens, turnip greens, mustard greens, kale, dark green leafy vegetables, broccoli, almonds, cheese, tofu, corn tortillas, legumes (dried beans), calcium-fortified soy milk, and calcium-fortified orange juice. The following list ranks the best food sources of calcium, with the amount of calcium in parentheses.

Calcium All-Stars

- yogurt, nonfat plain, 8 oz. (452 mg)
- orange juice or grapefruit juice, calcium-fortified, 1 cup (300–400 mg)
- yogurt, fruit-flavored, 8 oz. (314 mg)
- milk, low-fat or skim, 1 cup (300 mg)
- tofu, packaged with calcium, ½ cup firm (258 mg)
- cheddar cheese, lower-fat, 1 oz. (200 mg)
- salmon with bones, canned, 3 oz. (181 mg)
- Parmesan cheese, grated, 2 tablespoons (138 mg)
- cottage cheese, low-fat, ½ cup (69–100 mg)
- broccoli, chopped, boiled, 1 cup (72 mg)

Magnesium

Studies have shown that populations that eat a magnesium-rich diet have lower rates of hypertension. "Hard water," in addition to being high in calcium, also contains high amounts of magnesium, and people who live in hard-water regions have much lower rates of hypertension-related disease. In one review of 30 studies from 12 countries, investigators found that people whose diet contains high amounts of magnesium have less hypertension than those who eat a diet low in magnesium. A study of 12 districts in South Africa revealed that as the concentration of magnesium in the drinking water got lower and lower, the rate of hypertension got higher and higher. Even animals fed a diet low in magnesium tended to develop high blood pressure.

Magnesium helps keep blood pressure healthy by interacting with calcium to open up the blood vessels.

The government's recommended daily allowance (RDA) of magnesium is 400 milligram per day, but the average American eats only half that amount. This dietary deficiency may account in part for the prevalence of hypertension in our society. Eating the DASH diet ensures you get 500 milligrams of magnesium in your diet every day. We decided on this amount by looking at studies showing how much magnesium is in the diet of populations that tend to have healthy blood pressure.

Nuts are a major dietary source of magnesium. Other sources include legumes, such as black beans, black-eyed peas, and pinto beans; peanut butter; whole grains; dark green leafy vegetables, such as spinach; cereals, such as brown rice, wheat germ, wheat bran, and oatmeal; seafood, such as bluefish, carp, cod, flounder, halibut, herring, mackerel, ocean perch, shrimp, and swordfish; and bananas.

How Potassium, Calcium, and Magnesium Combine to Lower Blood Pressure

When we reviewed studies of the effects of potassium, calcium, and magnesium on blood pressure, certain things became clear. Yes, populations that eat diets high in these key minerals tend to have healthy blood pressure, but scientists have not been able to consistently reproduce this beneficial relationship in research studies. Even when studies showed that minerals did appear to work to lower blood pressure, the reductions were minimal. Part of the problem turned out to be that most of these studies were done using mineral pill supplements, and we've come to understand that minerals aren't as effective at lowering blood pressure when consumed in this form. It appears that minerals are much more effective at lowering blood pressure when they are eaten in whole foods, possibly because of the presence of other beneficial minerals in those foods that increase their effectiveness.

What this information suggested to us was that, to be effective at lowering blood pressure, potassium, calcium, and magnesium needed to be combined and consumed in a diet of whole foods.

How certain minerals combine to lower blood pressure

and why they work better together as part of a whole-food diet are highly complex and not yet well-understood processes. But given the success of the DASH diet—an eating plan that emphasizes whole foods rich in key minerals thought to lower blood pressure, not pills containing individual concentrations or combinations of these key minerals—we believe this is indeed what happens.

Fiber Matters Too

Despite the uncertainty about fiber, we believe it is an important part of the DASH diet. Numerous observational studies have shown that populations that eat a diet high in fiber—especially soluble fiber—are less likely to have hypertension than those that do not.

Fiber is an undigestable complex carbohydrate found in plants. This substance is divided into two types according to its physical characteristics and how it affects your body: water-insoluble and water-soluble.

You should eat both types of fiber, because each functions differently and provides different health benefits. Imagine insoluble fiber as being crunchy and soluble fiber as sticky. We are quite clear on what insoluble fiber does. It "bulks up" waste and moves it through the bowel more rapidly, preventing constipation and colon problems, such as diverticulosis, irritable bowel syndrome, and possibly colon cancer. The job of soluble fiber is more complex. These sticky gums and pectins regulate various processes in your body, including cholesterol and blood sugar production. They also may influence blood pressure, although how is not well understood.

Again, to say categorically that fiber is a major antihypertensive factor based on studies showing that populations that eat a high-fiber diet have lower rates of hypertension may be misguided, because many foods rich in soluble fiber, such as fruits and vegetables, are also high in other important nutri-

---

What Foods Supply Which Fiber?

Insoluble Fiber: Fruits, vegetables, dried beans, wheat bran, seeds, popcorn, brown rice, and whole-grain products, such as breads, cereals, and pasta

Soluble Fiber: Fruits, such as apples, oranges, pears, peaches, and grapes; vegetables, seeds, oat bran, dried beans, oatmeal, barley, and rye

---

ents, including potassium, calcium, and magnesium. The results of interventional studies to test the effect of fiber on blood pressure have been inconsistent. When such studies did achieve beneficial results, the results were modest.

Most nutritionists recommend a diet containing 20 to 35 grams of fiber a day. The average American diet contains barely half this amount, which may explain the rise in the incidence of several killer diseases, including hypertension. The DASH diet provides 30 grams of fiber a day.

Sources of Fiber

Food	Serving Size	Total Fiber (grams)
Legumes (cooked)		
Kidney beans	½ cup	6.7
Pinto beans	½ cup	6.7
Vegetables (cooked)		
Broccoli, chopped	½ cup	2.6
Brussels sprouts	½ cup	3.8
Spinach	½ cup	2.1
Zucchini, sliced	½ cup	1.6
Fruits (raw)		
Apple	1 medium	3.6

Grapefruit	½ medium	1.8
Grapes	1 cup	1.1
Orange	1 medium	2.9
Prunes	6 medium	8.0
Grains		
Brown rice (cooked)	½ cup	1.8
Corn flakes	1 ounce	0.3
Oat bran (dry)	⅓ cup	4.4
Oatmeal (dry)	⅓ cup	2.8
Shredded wheat	½ cup	3.5
White bread	1 slice	0.4
Whole-wheat bread	1 slice	2.1

Appendix B

———————————/\———————————

A Formula to Calculate
Your Daily Calorie Intake

On pages 78–79 there is a table you can use to estimate your daily calorie intake. But if you want to do the math yourself, you can use the following three-step formula.

1. Calculate Your Basic Metabolic Rate (BMR)

a. First, divide your body weight in pounds by 2.2 to find your weight in kilograms.
b. Then multiply your kilogram body weight by 1 if you are a man, by 0.9 if you are a woman.
c. Multiply the result by 24 for the number of hours in the day.

Sample Worksheet

A 180-pound man's BMR is 180 ÷ 2.2 × 1 × 24, or 1,964 calories per day.
A 150-pound woman's BMR is 150 ÷ 2.2 × 0.9 × 24, or 1,473 calories per day.

This tells you what your calorie expenditure is when you are at rest, known as your "BMR" (basal metabolic rate), which doesn't take into consideration how active you are.

2. Calculate Your Activity Quotient

a. Start by checking off the activities you engage in from the following list:

Activity	Points
1. Gardening or other moderate lawn work, several hours every week	1
2. Walking for exercise or recreation three or more times per week	①
3. Walking to and from work or shopping (at least ½ mile each way)	①
4. Job/household routine (select only one of the next three):	
a. Office work, light physical activity, or household chores	0
b. Farm work, being on your feet most of the day, or equivalent activities	4
c. Heavy physical activity (shoveling, lifting, etc.)	⑨
5. Fishing an average of once a week or more (sitting on the dock does not count)	1
6. Vigorous dancing every week for an hour or more	1
7. Playing golf at least once a week during the season (walking the course, no carts)	2
8. Using the stairs instead of elevators or escalators	1
9. Using exercise to relax from life pressures	①

10. Calisthenics (sit-ups, push-ups, etc.)   3
    at least 10 minutes at a time, twice a week
    or more
11. Yoga, stretching, or equivalent activities   2
    on a regular basis
12. Recreational sports: tennis, handball,
    badminton, Frisbee, etc. (select only one
    of the next three):
    a. Once a week   2
    b. Twice a week   4
    c. Three times a week or more   7
13. Vigorous exercise, such as jogging,
    swimming, mountain biking, in-line
    skating, squash, or the equivalent, for
    at least 20 continuous minutes per
    session (select only one of the next three):
    a. Once a week   3
    b. Twice a week   5
    c. Three times a week or more   10

b. Now add up the points for each activity to calculate your
   activity quotient.

Points	Activity Quotient
0–1	1.0
2–10	1.3
11–20	1.5
21–30	1.7
31–40	1.9

3. Multiply Your BMR by Your Activity Quotient

Now multiply your BMR (from number 1 above) by your activity quotient (1.0 to 1.9). This gives you your approximate daily calorie requirement.

Sample Worksheet

Let's say the 180-pound male from number 1 has an activity quotient of 1.5. Multiply his BMR (1,964 calories) by 1.5 to find that he needs 2,946 calories a day to *maintain* his present weight. Consuming more calories will result in weight (fat) gain, and consuming fewer calories will result in weight (fat) loss.

Appendix C

———————⋀———————

A Formula to Calculate
Your Body Mass Index (BMI)

The easy-to-use table on pages 48–49 can be used to find your body mass index (BMI), a number that defines your weight as "normal/healthy," "underweight," "overweight," or "obese." You can also calculate your BMI using the following formula.

1. Multiply your weight in pounds by 703.
2. Determine your height in inches.
3. Multiply your height by itself.
4. Divide the answer from step 1 by the answer from step 3.

Your answer is your BMI.

Example: As an example, we are going to use an individual who is 5 feet 5 inches tall and weighs 150 pounds.

$150 \times 703 = 105,450$
$5'5" = 65$ inches
$65 \times 65 = 4,225$
$105,450/4,225 = 24.9$ BMI

If Your BMI Is . . .	*You Are Considered . . .*
less than 20	underweight
20–24.9	normal/healthy weight
25–30	overweight
more than 30	obese

Appendix D

Scientific Articles
About the DASH Diet

Some of you may be interested in reading the scientific articles that the DASH group and others have written about the DASH diet. Below is a list of many such articles. More are being published all the time, so we apologize that this list is not complete and current. If you are interested in a more current list and you have access to Medline searching (on the Web at http://igm.nlm.nih.gov/), search on the term "DASH Diet." This should provide references to almost all the published literature.

Articles by Members of the DASH Team

Sacks FM, Obarzanek E, Windhauser MM, Svetkey LP, Vollmer WM, McCullough M, Karanja N, Lin PH, Steele P, Proschan MA, et al. Rationale and design for the Dietary Approaches to Stop Hypertension trial (DASH). A multicenter controlled-feeding study of dietary patterns to lower blood pressure. Ann Epidemiol. 1995 Mar; 5(2):108–18.

Appel LJ, Moore TJ, Obarzanek E, Vollmer WM, Svetkey LP, Sacks FM, Bray GA, Vogt TM, Cutler JA, Windhauser MM, Lin PH, Karanja N. A clinical trial of the effects of dietary patterns on blood pressure. DASH Collaborative

Research Group. N Engl J Med. 1997 Apr 17; 336(16): 1117–24.

Moore TJ for the DASH Steering Committee. Letter to editor. Science. 1998; 282:1049–50.

DASH Collaborative Research Group. The effect of dietary patterns on blood pressure: results from the Dietary Approaches to Stop Hypertension (DASH) clinical trial. Current Concepts in Hypertension. 1998 Nov; 2:4–5.

Miller ER 3rd, Appel LJ, Risby TH. Effect of dietary patterns on measures of lipid peroxidation: results from a randomized clinical trial. Circulation. 1998 Dec 1; 98(22):2390–5.

Obarzanek E, Moore TJ. Foreword: Using feeding studies to test the efficacy of dietary interventions: Lessons from the Dietary Approaches to Stop Hypertension Trial. J Amer Dietetic Assoc 1999; 99:S9–10.

Vogt TM, Appel LJ, Obarzanek E, Moore TJ, Vollmer WM, Svetkey LP, Sacks FM, Bray GA, Cutler JA, Windhauser MM, Lin PH, Karanja NM, for the DASH Collaborative Research Group. Dietary Approaches to Stop Hypertension: rationale, design and methods. J Amer Dietetic Assoc 1999; 99:S12–18.

Karanja NM, Obarzanek E, Lin PH, McCullough ML, Phillips KM, Swain JF, Champagne CM, Hoben KP, for the DASH Collaborative Research Group. Descriptive characteristics of the dietary patterns used in the Dietary Approaches to Stop Hypertension trial. J Amer Dietetic Assoc 1999; 99:S19–27.

Karanja NM, McCullough ML, Kumanyika SK, Pedula KL, Windhauser MM, Obarzanek E, Lin PH, Champagne CM, Swain J, for the DASH Collaborative Research Group. Pre-enrollment diets of Dietary Approaches to Stop Hypertension trial participants. J Amer Dietetic Assoc 1999; 99:S28–34.

Harsha DW, Pao-Hwa L, Obarzanek E, Karanja NM, Moore TJ, Caballero B. Dietary Approaches to Stop Hypertension: A summary of results. J Amer Dietetic Assoc 1999; 99:S35–39.

Lin PH, Windhauser MM, Plaisted CS, Hoben KP, McCullough ML, Obarzanek E, for the DASH Collaborative Research Group. The linear index model for establishing nutrient goals in the Dietary Approaches to Stop Hypertension trial. J Amer Dietetic Assoc 1999; 99: S40–44.

McCullough ML, Karanja NM, Lin PH, Obarzanek E, Phillips KM, Laws RL, Vollmer WM, O'Connor EA, Champagne CM, Windhauser MM, for the DASH Collaborative Research Group. Comparison of 4 nutrient databases with chemical composition data from the Dietary Approaches to Stop Hypertension trial. J Amer Dietetic Assoc 1999; 99: S45–53.

Swain JF, Windhauser MM, Hoben KP, Evans MA, McGee BB, Steele PD, for the DASH Collaborative Research Group. Menu design and selection for multicenter controlled feeding studies: process used in the Dietary Approaches to Stop Hypertension trial. J Amer Dietetic Assoc 1999; 99:S54–59.

Phillips KM, Stewart KK, Karanja NM, Windhauser MM, Champagne CM, Swain JF, Lin PH, Evans MA, for the DASH Collaborative Research Group. Validation of diet composition for the Dietary Approaches to Stop Hypertension trial. J Amer Dietetic Assoc 1999; 99: S60–68.

Appel LJ, Vollmer WM, Obarzanek E, Aicher KM, Conlin PR, Kennedy BM, Charleston JB, Reams PM, for the DASH Collaborative Research Group. Recruitment and baseline characteristics of participants in the Dietary Approaches to Stop Hypertension trial. J Amer Dietetic Assoc 1999; 99:S69–75.

Windhauser MM, Evans MA, McCullough ML, Swain JF, Lin PH, Hoben KP, Plaisted CS, Karanja NM, Vollmer WM, for the DASH Collaborative Research Group. Dietary adherence in the Dietary Approaches to Stop Hypertension trial. J Amer Dietetic Assoc 1999; 99:S76–83.

Plaisted CS, Lin PH, Ard JD, McClure ML, Svetkey LP. The effects of dietary patterns on quality of life: a substudy of the Dietary Approaches to Stop Hypertension trial. J Amer Dietetic Assoc 1999; 99:S84–89.

Windhauser MM, Ernst DB, Karanja NM, Crawford SW, Redican SE, Swain JF, Karimbakas JM, Champagne CM, Hoben KP, Evans MA, for the DASH Collaborative Research Group. Translating the Dietary Approaches to Stop Hypertension diet from research to practice: dietary and behavior change techniques. J Amer Dietetic Assoc 1999; 99: S90–95.

Svetkey LP, Sacks FM, Obarzanek E, Vollmer WM, Appel LJ, Lin PH, Karanja NM, Harsha DW, Bray GA, Aickin M, Proschan MA, Windhauser MM, Swain JF, McCarron PB, Rhodes DG, Laws RL, for the DASH-Sodium Collaborative Research Group. The DASH diet, sodium intake and blood pressure trial (DASH-sodium): rationale and design. J Amer Dietetic Assoc 1999; 99:S96–104.

Sacks FM, Appel LJ, Moore TJ, Obarzanek E, Vollmer WM, Svetkey LP, Bray GA, Vogt TM, Cutler JA, Windhauser MM, Lin PH, Karanja N. A dietary approach to prevent hypertension: a review of the Dietary Approaches to Stop Hypertension (DASH) Study. Clin Cardiol. 1999 Jul; 22(7 Suppl):III 6–10.

Appel LJ. Nonpharmacologic therapies that reduce blood pressure: a fresh perspective. Clin Cardiol. 1999 Jul; 22(7 Suppl):III 1–5. Review.

Svetkey LP, Simons-Morton D, Vollmer WM, Appel LJ, Conlin PR, Ryan DH, Ard J, Kennedy BM. Effects of dietary patterns on blood pressure: subgroup analysis of the Dietary Approaches to Stop Hypertension (DASH) randomized clinical trial. Arch Intern Med. 1999 Feb; 159(3): 285–93.

Moore TJ, Vollmer WM, Appel LJ, Sacks FM, Svetkey LP,

Vogt TM, Conlin PR, Simons-Morton DG, Carter-Edwards L, Harsha DW. Effect of dietary patterns on ambulatory blood pressure: results from the Dietary Approaches to Stop Hypertension (DASH) trial. Hypertension. 1999 Sep; 34(3):472–77.

Appel LJ, Miller ER 3rd, Jee SH, Stolzenberg-Solomon R, Lin PH, Erlinger T, Nadeau MR, Selhub J. Effect of dietary patterns on serum homocysteine: results of a randomized, controlled feeding study. Circulation. 2000 Aug 22; 102(8):852–57.

Conlin PR, Chow D, Miller ER 3rd, Svetkey LP, Lin PH, Harsha DW, Moore TJ, Sacks FM, Appel LJ. The effect of dietary patterns on blood pressure control in hypertensive patients: results from the Dietary Approaches to Stop Hypertension (DASH) trial. Am J Hypertens. 2000 Sep; 13(9):949–55.

Sacks FM, Svetkey LP, Vollmer WM, Appel LJ, Bray GA, Harsha D, Obarzanek E, Conlin PR, Miller ER, Simons-Morton DG, Karanja N, Lin PH, Aickin M, Most-Windhauser M, Moore TJ, Proschan MA, Cutler JA. Effects on blood pressure of reduced dietary sodium and the Dietary Approaches to Stop Hypertension (DASH) diet. N Engl J Med 2001; 344:3–10.

Articles by Other Investigators

(No authors listed) The DASH diet. It may benefit your blood pressure, and more. Mayo Clin Health Lett. 1998 Apr; 16(4):7.

Zemel MB. Dietary pattern and hypertension: the DASH study. Dietary Approaches to Stop Hypertension. Nutr Rev. 1997 Aug; 55(8):303–5. Review.

Tucker K. Dietary patterns and blood pressure in African Americans. Nutr Rev. 1999 Nov; 57(11):356–58. Review.

Kolasa KM. Dietary Approaches to Stop Hypertension

(DASH) in clinical practice: a primary care experience. Clin Cardiol. 1999 July; 22(7 Suppl):III 16–22. Review.

Fraser GE. Nut consumption, lipids, and risk of a coronary event. Clin Cardiol. 1999 July; 22(7 Suppl):III 11–15. Review.

K Hermansen. Diet, blood pressure and hypertension. Br J Nutr. 2000 Mar; 83 Suppl 1:S113–19. Review.

Miller GD, DiRienzo DD, Reusser ME, McCarron DA. Benefits of dairy product consumption on blood pressure in humans: a summary of the biomedical literature. J Am Coll Nutr. 2000 Apr; 19 (2 Suppl):147S–164S. Review.

Index

Not sure what to read next?

Visit Pocket Books online at
www.simonsays.com

Reading suggestions for
you and your reading group
New release news
Author appearances
Online chats with your favorite writers
Special offers
Order books online
And much, much more!

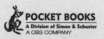

POCKET BOOKS
A Division of Simon & Schuster
A CBS COMPANY

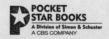

POCKET STAR BOOKS
A Division of Simon & Schuster
A CBS COMPANY

13456

More than 50 million Americans suffer from high blood pressure, and most of them control it by taking prescription drugs with potentially dangerous side effects; and nearly 24 million Americans have diabetes. But there is a natural and affordable alternative for managing these potentially deadly conditions, reducing your risk of heart failure, stroke, and kidney disease, and achieving the best health of your life: the DASH (Dietary Approaches to Stop Hypertension) diet. Developed by a world-class team of doctors and nutritionists, the DASH diet gives you:

- Complete and balanced nutrition for safe short-term and long-term weight loss

- A scientifically proven approach to managing diabetes and heart disease *without* prescription medication

- A hearty and healthful selection of DASH menus, recipes, and grocery lists

- DASH exercise programs for everyday living

- Key tools including calorie worksheets and a formula to calculate body mass

. . . and much more from this revolutionary program, which is recommended by the American Heart Association; the National Heart, Lung, and Blood Institute; the American Society for Hypertension; and other leading medical authorities.

"YOU CAN'T GO WRONG WITH THE DASH DIET."
–Andrew Weil, M.D.

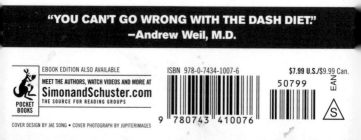